# THE 2023 COMPLETE FOODS LISTS FOR DIABETES

## PRACTICAL TOOLS & MEAL PLANNING GUIDE — WITH 1300+ FOOD RANKED BY THEIR GI, GL VALUES

### DR. H. MAHER

❀ Created with Vellum

# CONTENTS

Part IX
THE WORST FOODS TO EAT (HIGH GLYCEMIC
LOAD FOOD)

meats, rich in fresh fruits and vegetables, dark leafy greens, whole grain cereals, and legumes. It emphasizes unprocessed or minimally processed fatty foods as fat sources, such as nuts, seeds, olive oil, fatty fish, white meat, eggs, fermented plant food, and fermented dairy products.

Using the glycemic load to rank carbohydrate-containing foods according to their effects on glycemia is the mainstay of the balanced diet for diabetes. It supplies your body with low glycemic, unprocessed, or minimally processed foods, with little to no unhealthy added constituents. Therefore, you don't have to focus on calorie, protein, fat, or carb counting. Instead, you have to create a diabetes-friendly eating plan and check out the resources in this book for foods, guidelines, and tools to make it easier to eat balanced, so your blood sugar remains in your target range as much as possible.

---

In addition to extensive diabetes-friendly foods lists chosen based on their glycemic load values, you'll also learn why and how to:

1. **plan for regular, balanced meals** to prevent high or low blood glucose levels.
2. **choose low glycemic load foods and beverages** more often to maintain your blood sugar under control.
3. **use the plate method to plan your meals quickly.**
4. **stay hydrated.** Drinking enough water helps your body remove excess sugar through urine.
5. **choose healthy cooking methods,** such as broiling, roasting, stir-frying, or grilling.
6. **choose fresh or frozen unprocessed foods** or canned foods with no added sugar or salt.
7. **increase your olive oil consumption** as it lowers glucose levels, LDL (low-density lipoprotein), and triglycerides.
8. **choose foods with no added sugar.** Added sugars include

brown sugar, honey, cane juice, fructose, dextrose, sucrose, lactose, corn sweetener, and corn syrup.

9. **exclude Trans-Fats containing Foods.** Trans-fats include margarine, vegetable shortening, french fries, Nondairy creamer, and frozen pizza.

10. **avoid highly processed foods**. Examples of ultra-processed foods include sugary drinks, flavored potato chips, poultry nuggets and sticks, and fish nuggets.

# PART I
# UNDERSTANDING DIABETES

# WHAT IS DIABETES?

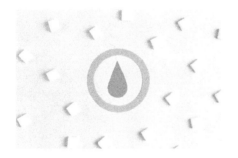

Diabetes is a chronic metabolic illness marked by unsuitable hyperglycemia due to a lack of insulin or insulin resistance. Its adverse health effects can seriously reduce life expectancy significantly by ten years. Several lifestyle factors and dietary habits affect type 1 and type 2 diabetes incidence, such as types and amounts of food ingested, weight gain, obesity, physical activity, watching TV or sedentary time, and sleep quality.

Diabetes mellitus is a chronic endocrine illness that influences how the body utilizes food for energy and is marked by abnormally high blood glucose levels. Insulin — the hormone made by the pancreas— allows glucose to get into body cells to provide energy. When blood sugar levels rise after eating, your pancreas releases sufficient insulin into the blood. Insulin then reduces blood sugar to keep it in the normal range. In people with diabetes, the pancreas cannot perform this fundamental function, or the body's cells do not respond adequately to the insulin produced. The blood sugar level then increases, and sugar accumulates in the body and becomes toxic to the vital organs. Having a high glucose level in the blood can cause severe health problems. It can irreversibly cause severe damage to the eyes, kidneys, heart, and nerves. There are three main types of diabetes:

## TYPE 1 DIABETES

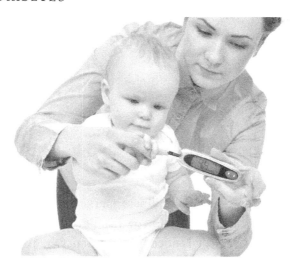

Type 1 diabetes mellitus (DM) is a chronic autoimmune disease characterized by the immune system's destruction of insulin-producing pancreatic *beta* cells. The body will no longer make insulin due to irreversible damage to the insulin-producing cells. Without insulin hormones, glucose can not get into the body's cells, and the blood glucose increases above normal. People with type 1 must inject daily

4

insulin doses and follow a strict diet to stay alive and prevent severe adverse effects. Type 1 diabetes generally appears in children and young adults but may occur at any age.

In 2016, the FDA—Food and Drug Administration approved the artificial pancreas to replace manual blood glucose checking and the injection of insulin shots. These automated devices act like your real pancreas in controlling blood sugar and releasing insulin when the patient's blood sugar becomes too high. The artificial pancreas also releases a small flow of insulin continuously.

**Risk Factors**

Type 1 diabetes has diverse risk factors. Some are still under investigation and would bring a complete picture of the subject. Known risk factors include:

- **family history of type 1 diabetes**: The risk of developing type 1 diabetes significantly increases if you have a parent affected by type 1 diabetes. The risk is even higher if you have a brother or sister diagnosed with type 1 diabetes.
- **ethnicity**: Observational studies have shown that in the United States, white people have a raised risk of developing type 1 diabetes than African American, Hispanic or Latino people.
- **age**: type 1 diabetes generally occurs at an early age. However, you can get it at any age. The prevalence and incidence of type 1 diabetes in teens or young adults are increasing yearly.
- **viral infections**: recent studies suggest that some viruses, such as coxsackievirus B, mumps virus, and cytomegalovirus, can trigger the development of type 1 diabetes by deregulating the immune system.
- **vitamin D deficiency**: poor vitamin D status is linked with an increased risk of developing type 1 diabetes due to the essential role of vitamin D in regulating the immune system. An adequate vitamin D status plays a protective role on the

immune system and is linked to decreased risk of type 1 diabetes.

**Symptoms of Type 1 Diabetes**

Type 1 diabetes symptoms can develop abruptly in just a few weeks and can be severe. Symptoms and signs include

- frequent thirst and urination
- increased hunger
- fruity-smelling, which indicates diabetic ketoacidosis (DKA), a severe complication of type 1 diabetes.
- unexplained weight loss
- blurred vision
- stomach pains
- nausea and vomiting
- frequent urinary infections
- fatigue and tiredness

Unfortunately, type 1 DM is chronic immune-mediated and remains incurable. However, you can lower the risk of complications and improve its management by adhering to the glycemic load lifestyle.

---

TYPE 2 DIABETES

**Prediabetes**. Even if a person is not sick, he may suffer from prediabetes without knowing it. This term refers to an intermediate stage characterized by an abnormally higher blood glucose level than usual. That represents a warning signal that informs people with prediabetes diagnosis that they are at increased risk of type 2 diabetes mellitus if they don't take appropriate and urgent action, especially if they have other risk factors, including:

- overweight,
- obesity,
- sedentary lifestyle,
- high blood pressure.

Type 2 diabetes (T2DM) is the most prevalent type of diabetes (8 to 10 times more than type 1 diabetes). Its prevalence and incidence are increasing worldwide. It is estimated that the prevalence of type 2 diabetes is nearly 10%, including diagnosed and undiagnosed. According to recent statistics, the number of people affected by diabetes increased from 108 million in 1980 to 536 million in 2021.

T2DM is a chronic metabolic disease that occurs when the pancreas does not release enough insulin to regulate blood sugar and/or when the body becomes unable effectively use the insulin it makes. The body cannot use glucose or sugar as fuel and regulate blood sugar which causes uncontrolled high blood sugar or hyperglycemia. Type 2 diabetes is induced by several factors, including lifestyle factors, strict diets, overweight, obesity, Hyperthyroidism, and genes.

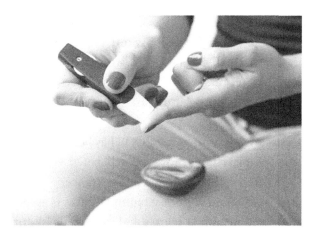

Type 2 diabetes (DM) can develop at any age. However, it's more common after the age of forty-five.

**Risk Factors**

Type 2 Diabetes has diverse risk factors. Some are controllable such as being overweight, obese, or vitamin D deficient, and others are uncontrollable such as age and family history of diabetes. Known risk factors include:

- **overweight and obesity**: are two main predictors of developing type 2 diabetes. People who are obese are at elevated risk of developing diabetes and experiencing its complications. Fortunately, obesity and overweight are reversible through an adequate diet, such as the glycemic load.
- **type 2 diabetes family history:** The risk of developing T2DM increases if you have a parent affected by it.
- **ethnicity**: Observational studies have shown that in the United States, T2DM is more prevalent in African American, Hispanic or Latino, American Indian, or Asian American people.
- **age 45 or older**: type 2 diabetes generally occurs at the of forty-five. However, you can develop it even in your childhood.
- **high blood pressure (hypertension)**: type 2 diabetes and hypertension usually co-occur. However, new studies suggest that high blood pressure significantly raises the risk of developing cardiovascular diseases and type 2 diabetes if not treated properly.
- **polycystic ovary syndrome:** PCOS has been recently identified as a risk factor for type 2 diabetes. Women affected by PCOS often suffer from insulin resistance,
- **vitamin D deficiency**: poor vitamin D status is associated with impaired insulin D release and increased risk for developing insulin resistance and/or metabolic syndrome. Adequate vitamin D status is shown to improve insulin sensitivity and improve type 2 diabetes management.

## SYMPTOMS OF TYPE 2 DIABETES

Type 2 diabetes symptoms and signs develop slowly and can take years to develop. Some patients don't notice any symptoms at all until they get diagnosed. Type 2 diabetes generally begins at an adult age, though more and more people are developing it at a young age due to excess sugar consumption. Because symptoms are hard to identify or take longer to develop, it's crucial to be aware of the risk factors and visit your doctor accordingly.

Symptoms and signs of T2DM include:

- abnormal and intense thirst
- frequent urination
- exaggerated hunger
- unexplained and sudden weight loss
- irritability
- blurred vision
- dry mouth
- stomach pains
- nausea and vomiting
- poorly healing wounds
- frequent urinary infections
- fatigue and tiredness

## GESTATIONAL DIABETES

Gestational diabetes is the high blood sugar that occurs during pregnancy in women who did not have diabetes before becoming pregnant. Gestational diabetes is more frequent in the second or third trimester but can occur at any time of pregnancy and usually disappears after giving birth.

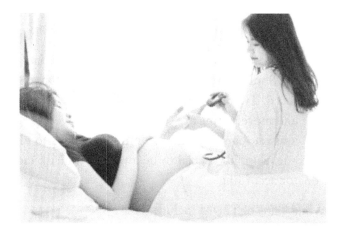

Women diagnosed with it are at higher risk of developing T2DM later in life, particularly for women with favoring factors (obesity, imbalanced diet, sedentary lifestyle, metabolic syndrome).

In most cases, gestational diabetes does not induce symptoms and goes silent and unnoticed. When symptoms are present, they may be misperceived as pregnancy aches and discomfort. Symptoms of gestational diabetes are the same as type 2 diabetes and include:

- intense thirst
- increased hunger
- unusual fatigue
- stomach pains
- nausea and vomiting
- more frequent urination
- urinary infections
- headaches

If you are pregnant, you may get tested for diabetes between 24 and 28 weeks of pregnancy.

For most women affected by gestational diabetes, **the diabetes is reversible and goes away soon after delivery**. However, women who have experienced hyperglycemia during their pregnancy should have their blood sugar levels regularly monitored due to the high risk of developing type 2 diabetes among this population.

---

**Common Symptoms of Diabetes**

Diabetes symptoms may vary depending on the level of blood sugar. Some people with prediabetes or type 2 diabetes may initially not experience frank symptoms. Conversely, with type 1 diabetes, symptoms come on quickly and severely.

Bellow a list of common symptoms and signs of type 1 and type 2 diabetes and gestational diabetes:

- increased craving
- frequent urination
- excessive hunger
- weight loss
- ketones in the urine
- fatigue and tiredness
- increased irritability
- blurred vision
- slow healing wounds and cuts
- frequent infections

# INSULIN RESISTANCE AND PREDIABETES

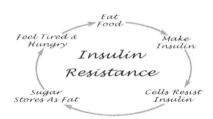

Insulin is a polypeptide hormone that controls and regulates the absorption of sugar by body cells and maintains the level of sugar present in the blood at a healthy level. This hormone is produced by the β cells of the pancreas. When you eat, food moves to your stomach and intestines to be broken down into micronutrients absorbed and transported by our bloodstream. The pancreas produces insulin through its β cells and releases it into the bloodstream when we eat to allow body cells, including muscles and other cells, to absorb and transform sugar (glucose) into energy throughout the body.

Insulin also signals to the liver, muscle, and adipocytes (fat cells) to store the excess glucose for further use. Extra sugar is stored in 3 ways:

- In muscle tissues as glycogen.
- In the liver as glycogen.
- In adipose tissue (fat reserves of the body) in the form of triglycerides—which are fat molecules that store energy

## INSULIN RESISTANCE

Insulin resistance is a serious and silent health condition that occurs when cells in your muscles, liver, and body fat start ignoring the signal that the insulin hormone is sending out to transfer sugar out of the bloodstream and put it into your body cells. As insulin resistance develops, the body reacts by producing more and more insulin to lower blood sugar.

Over time, the β cells in the pancreas working hard to make a higher supply of insulin can no longer provide more and more insulin. Your blood sugar may reflect the pancreas' failure to maintain the level in the healthy range, and your blood sugar rises, showing pre-diabetes or, at worst, type 2 diabetes.

Insulin resistance is silent and presents no symptoms in the first stage of its development. The symptoms appear later when the condition worsens, and the pancreas cannot produce sufficient insulin to maintain your blood glucose within the normal range. When this occurs, the symptoms may be severe, including metabolic syndrome, polycystic ovary syndrome (PCOS), and various types of diabetes.

Fortunately, it is possible to lower the effects of insulin resistance and boost your insulin sensitivity by following a low-glycemic load diet.

Thus, for many of you, following a low-glycemic diet goes beyond weight-loss management and target the management of particular health condition sensitive to such kind of diet and particularly those related to insulin resistance like:

- Excessive hunger
- Lethargy or tiredness
- Difficulty concentrating
- Brain fog
- Waist weight gain
- High blood pressure

## CAN INSULIN RESISTANCE BE REDUCED OR REVERSED?

Fortunately, It is possible to lower the effects of insulin resistance and boost your insulin sensitivity by following some effective methods, including:

- Low glycemic load diet
- Low carbohydrate and high-fat diet
- Low-calorie diets
- Weight loss surgery
- Regular exercise in combination with healthy diets

These methods have a similar way of working. They all reduce the daily glucose intake drastically, lower the body's need for insulin, reduce insulin spikes in the bloodstream, promote weight loss and prevent weight gain.

# DIABETES TESTS & DIAGNOSIS

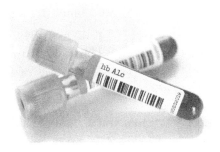

Diabetes, prediabetes, and gestational diabetes are diagnosed through blood tests which show if your blood sugar is too high. You'll need to get your blood glucose tested to determine if you have prediabetes, type 1, type 2 diabetes, or gestational diabetes. Refrain from self-diagnosing if you think you might have diabetes. Commercially available testing tools like blood glucose meter cannot diagnose diabetes. If you have symptoms of diabetes, you should ask your doctor to get your blood sugar tested. Testing is quick and straightforward and allows your doctor to screen for diabetes sooner and work with you to manage diabetes efficiently and prevent complications.

Your doctor will use the A1C test, the fasting plasma glucose (FPG) test, or the random plasma glucose RPG test to diagnose diabetes.

## THE A1C TEST AND DIABETES

The A1C test (also called hemoglobin A1C or HbA1c) is a blood test that measures the average levels of your blood sugar during the past two to three months. The A1C test is commonly used to diagnose prediabetes or type 2 diabetes risk. The A1C test is the primary tool for diabetes management, as patients use it to achieve their individual A1C goals.

**How does the test work?**

The A1C (HbA1c) test measures the sugar amount in your blood attached to hemoglobin—a protein in your red blood cells that carries oxygen. When sugar enters your bloodstream, it binds with hemoglobin. The A1C (HbA1c) test estimates the percentage of your red blood cells coated with glucose. Thus, a higher A1C (HbA1c) level indicates poor blood glucose control and warns of an elevated risk of developing severe diabetes complications.

If you have a diabetes condition, you should get an A1C (HbA1c) test at least twice a year to make sure diabetes is under close control and your blood glucose is in your target range.

**Interpreting the A1C results**

A normal A1C (HbA1c) level is under 5.7%. In healthy people, the normal range for the A1c (HbA1c) level is in the range of 4% to 5.6%

A level of A1C (HbA1c) in the range of 5.7-6.4% indicates prediabetes and a higher chance of developing diabetes.

A level of A1C (HbA1c) equal to or high than 6.5% indicates diabetes.

## THE FASTING PLASMA GLUCOSE TEST

The fasting blood sugar (FPG) test measures your blood sugar after an overnight 8 to 10 hours fast. It's a simple, safe, and quick way to screen for prediabetes, type1 and type 2 diabetes, or gestational diabetes. If you have a fasting blood sugar test scheduled, don't eat or drink for 8 to 12 hours before the test.

**How does the test work?**

When fasting, the pancreas hormone glucagon is stimulated and causes the liver to release glucose into the bloodstream, increasing blood glucose levels. If you don't have diabetes, your body will release insulin to burn excess glucose and rebalance the increased glucose levels. If you are affected by diabetes or prediabetes, your body cannot produce enough insulin or cannot use appropriately released insulin, causing blood glucose levels will remain high. Thus, a higher fasting plasma glucose level indicates poor blood glucose control and warns of an elevated risk of diabetes or prediabetes, depending on the test results.

**Interpreting the FPG results**

An FPG level less than or equal to 99 mg/dL is considered normal.

An FPG level of 100 **mg/dL (5.6 mmol/L)** to 125 mg/dL **(7 mmol/L)** indicates you have prediabetes and a higher risk of developing diabetes.

A fasting blood glucose level high than or equal to 126 mg/dL indicates you have diabetes.

## THE GLUCOSE TOLERANCE TEST

The Glucose Tolerance Test (OGTT) tests how your body moves glucose from the blood into the body's tissues. You then drink a liquid that contains glucose and get your blood measured. You'll fast overnight before taking the test and have your blood tested to assess your fasting blood glucose level.

Then you will drink the glucose-containing liquid and have your blood glucose level checked after 1 hour and 2 hours afterward.

**Interpreting the OGTT results**

At 2 hours test, a blood sugar level less than or equal to 140 mg/dL or lower is considered normal.

A blood sugar level in the range of 140-199 mg/dL indicates you have prediabetes and a higher risk of diabetes.

A blood sugar level high or equal to 200 mg/dL indicates you have diabetes.

## RANDOM BLOOD SUGAR TEST

The random blood sugar RPG test is sometimes used to diagnose diabetes when symptoms are present and when your doctor may need to screen for diabetes without waiting until you have fasted. You may take the RPG blood test at any time. An RPG blood glucose level high than or equal to 200 mg/dL indicates you have diabetes.

# DIABETES COMPLICATIONS

The complications of diabetes share a common origin: too much glucose in the blood. These complications happen in most individuals with uncontrolled type 1 and type 2 diabetes. A New body of evidence suggests that improved glycemic control significantly reduces the risk of microvascular complications and death from diabetes complications.

Over time, having an excess of sugar in your blood can cause complications ranging from mild to severe. Diabetes complications are often interrelated, share the same contributing causes, and combine in a dangerous way that may alter overall health. For example, nearly 50% of all patients diagnosed with type 2 diabetes have hypertension (high blood pressure), which may constrict and narrow the blood vessels throughout the body, including the nerves, the eyes, and the kidney. On the other side, having high glucose levels in your blood for a prolonged time can harm blood vessels that supply oxygen throughout your body, including the eyes, heart, kidneys, and brain. Damages that occur can lead to severe and long-term complications.

Diabetes also induces significant quantitative changes in the amount of circulating lipids characterized by an increase in triglycerides (a type of lipid in the blood), a reduction in HDL cholesterol (good), and an increase in LDL cholesterol (bad). These changes are linked with a raised risk of heart disease and stroke.

## THE MAIN COMPLICATIONS OF DIABETES

Diabetes complications are long-term problems that develop gradually. Diabetes complications can lead to severe damage if untreated.

- **diabetic retinopathy**. People affected by diabetes risk developing an eye disorder called retinopathy due to elevated high blood pressure. Retinopathy can affect patients' eyesight and cause partial vision loss and blindness.
- **diabetic foot ulcers**. Foot problems are severe diabetes complications that result from simultaneous actions, including damage to the nerve and impaired blood circulation. Nerve damages known as diabetic neuropathy combined with reduced blood flow affect the feeling in your feet and make it difficult for sores and cuts to heal. In some severe cases, gangrenes develop and can lead to amputation.
- **diabetic nephropathy**. This severe diabetes complication is common among type 1 and types 2 diabetes patients who poorly control their blood glucose. Over time, uncontrolled diabetes can lead to irreversible damage to blood vessel clusters that filter waste and extra water out of your blood, leading to kidney damage and kidney failure requiring the use of one of two blood purification techniques: hemodialysis and peritoneal dialysis. The evolution of diabetic nephropathy is also associated with other vascular complications of diabetes, either in the eyes (diabetic retinopathy) or the lower limbs (foot ulceration).
- **heart disease and stroke**. Over time, high blood glucose can harm vessels and nerves that control your heart and supply

oxygen to the brain and heart. Individuals affected by diabetes are at higher risk of cardiovascular diseases and strokes.

- **erectile dysfunction**. Prolonged and poor blood glucose control may damage nerves and small blood vessels controlling erection.
- **adhesive capsulitis of the shoulder.** People affected by diabetes are at greater risk of upper extremity joint damage, including capsulitis which is characterized by the inflammation of the joint capsule, a strong fibrous sheath surrounding the shoulder bones. Capsulitis occurs most often appears about 20 years after the onset of diabetes.
- **chronic inflammatory diseases**. Poorly controlled diabetes may cause damage to the whole body and trigger and worsen inflammation. In turn, inflammation causes and aggravates insulin resistance leading to much-elevated blood glucose levels.

# PART II
# KNOWING WHAT'S IN THE FOOD YOU EAT

# CARBOHYDRATES IN THE DIET

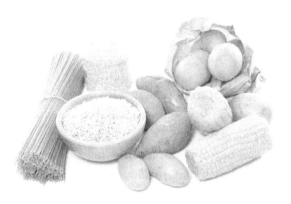

A diet rich in high-quality macronutrients is associated with a decreased risk of many chronic illnesses, including diabetes, chronic inflammation, cardiovascular disease, and high blood pressure. Strong evidence suggests that replacing foods of high energy density—high calories per weight of food—with foods of high nutrient density, such as vegetables, beans, and fruits, may help significantly improve glycemic control and promote weight loss.

Carbohydrates—or carbs are one of the three macronutrients in your diet, along with proteins and fats. Carbs play an essential role in the human body at every stage of life. They provide energy to all parts of your body (i.e., brain, heart, kidneys, muscles, liver, body's muscles), support the body's functions, promote good gut functioning (fiber), provide energy storage (as glycogen stored in the liver and muscles)

The consumption of high-quality carbohydrates is crucial for the success of long-term overall health, diabetes management, and weight loss.

## HOW DO HORMONES AFFECT WEIGHT AND DIABETES MANAGEMENT?

Before going deeper into the choice of healthy carbohydrates, we have to notice that you must achieve the following "Hormones balancing concepts":

- **getting and maintaining the insulin down** will allow you to increase your body's insulin sensitivity and reduce any form of insulin resistance.
- **avoiding spikes in insulin levels,** which are harmful to the pancreas and may induce insulin resistance, and increase cortisol levels —the hormone of stress— when the blood sugar decreases abruptly.
- **avoiding ultra-processed and high-processed foods** that compromise the guts' integrity and inhibit or reduce the release of leptin —the satiety hormone.
- **reducing the release of ghrelin**—the hunger hormone, by eating some nutrients that slow down the ghrelin release in the bloodstream.

## KNOWING HOW CARBOHYDRATES CAN WORK FOR YOU OR AGAINST YOU

All carbohydrates, whether low, moderate or high glycemic, follow the same metabolic pathway **that ensures a consistent energy supply to living cells by** breaking them down into simple sugar. They're then released into the bloodstream as glucose and enter the body's cells to provide them with energy with the help of insulin. The problem with blood sugar and subsequently with carbohydrates occurs when the blood sugar levels spike high throughout the day and frequently.

These spikes arise when you eat mostly high-glycemic foods or high-glycemic-load foods (a notion that refers to large portion sizes of carb-containing foods). Here comes the role of the glycemic index, which doesn't refer formally to a diet in that you must conform to strict rules, follow particular meal plans or eliminate some foods from your daily meals. Instead, it's a scientific method of identifying how carbohydrate affects blood sugar levels and measuring how slowly or quickly the carbohydrates in foods raise blood sugar. (please refer to part III for more details)

## TYPES OF CARBOHYDRATES IN YOUR DIET

The primary function of carbohydrates is to provide energy to the human body. Dietary carbohydrates can be divided into three major categories:

- sugars: Short-chain carbs found in foods such as fructose, glucose, sucrose, and galactose.
- starches: Long-chain of glucose molecules, which transform into glucose during digestion.
- fibers: are divided into soluble and insoluble.

Carbohydrates can also be divided according to their chemical composition into simple and complex carbs:

- complex carbohydrates are formed by sugar molecules linked together in complex and long chains. Complex carbs are found in vegetables, fruits, peas, beans, and whole grains and contain natural fiber. These types of food are healthy.
- simple carbohydrates are transformed quickly by the body and induce an increased sugar blood level. They are found in high amounts in processed foods and refined sugars.

Consumption of these carbs is associated with health problems like type 2 diabetes, obesity, and metabolism problems. Simple carbs foods are also deprived of essential nutrients and vitamins.

## CHOOSING THE BEST CARBOHYDRATES

Achieving your goals in weight loss, weight maintenance, or diabetes management depends on adapting your eating plan to make the insulin, leptin, and ghrelin hormones work for you. The quality of the carbohydrates you ingest is critical in adjusting the level of the hormones. For instance, low-quality carbs (high glycemic foods) are quickly digested and lead to blood sugar spikes, which will play against you and may cause weight gain, obesity, insulin resistance, and increased cortisol levels. Conversely, whole foods' soluble and insoluble fibers (low glycemic foods) are known to offset glucose conversion, prevent higher insulin supplies, and avoid irregular blood sugar variations that induce excess cortisol.

Low glycemic index Foods are known for releasing glucose in the blood slowly and regularly. Conversely, Foods that have a high glycemic index release glucose rapidly. Research suggests that foods with a low glycemic index are ideal for weight loss diets and foster weight loss, in addition to their positive effect on the pancreas (insulin release), eyes, and kidneys.

# UNDERSTANDING PROTEINS

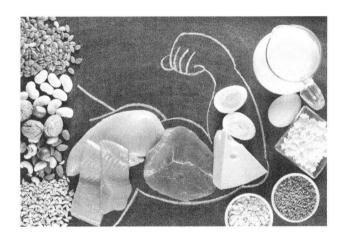

Proteins are, with carbohydrates and lipids, one of the three macronutrients in your diet. They consist of amino acids linked by peptide bonds. Proteins are essential for muscle and bone vitality and are involved in building and maintaining every cell in your body. They also intervene in many critical processes, such as creating and repairing tissues, building muscles, blood, hair, and skin, and producing hormones, enzymes, and other body chemicals.

Adequate protein consumption is essential for improving and maintaining optimal health during all stages of life. Unlike fats and carbs, the human body does not store protein, and you must eat an adequate amount to maintain overall health and promote optimal growth and body functions. In addition, eating enough protein reduces levels of ghrelin (the hunger hormone) and stimulates the production of the satiety hormones (PYY and GLP-1)

## GUIDELINES FOR INDIVIDUALIZED PROTEIN INTAKE

The Recommended Dietary Allowance (RDA) for protein is the minimum amount you need to satisfy your basic nutritional requirements. It corresponds to the minimum amount to maintain nitrogen balance (i.e., prevent you from getting sick). The RDA must be understood as the minimum you need to eat and is lower than what you should eat each day to maintain optimal health and achieve muscle growth. The RDA for protein to prevent deficiency is 0.8 g per kg of body weight, regardless of age. However, considering different parameters, it is recommended that people with diabetes and chronic kidney disease should aim for a protein intake of 0.8-1.0 grams per kg of body weight. People with diabetes and normal kidney functions should target a protein intake of 1.1-1.5 grams per kg.

## THE PROTEIN QUALITY

When looking for the best source of protein, the choice is based on two criteria: the PDCAA (Protein Digestibility Corrected Amino Acid) Score or the DIAA (Digestibility Indispensable Amino Acid) Score.

Animal-based foods Were found to provide excellent protein sources than plant proteins. Animal-based foods offer a complete composition of essential amino acids with higher bioavailability and digestibility (>90%).

## COLLAGEN, AN ESSENTIAL INGREDIENT

Collagen is a structural protein present in all the structures of the body, such as Ligaments, tendons, skin, hair, nails, discs, bones, and connective tissues. It represents nearly 30% of the total proteins in the body and ensures the cohesion, elasticity, and regeneration of these tissues. Collagen is present in three forms:

- type I is the most prevalent form of collagen in the body. Type 1 collagen is involved in the good structure of several tissues, including skin, tendons, and bone tissue.
- type II is the type of collagen that helps build connective tissues. It is present principally in cartilage, bone, and other connective tissues.
- type III is a major structural component in soft tissues, including muscles, blood vessels, the uterus, and the intestines.

During the normal aging process, your body begins to experience a decline in synthesizing collagen proteins. According to studies, this decline in collagen production starts around 30, at a rate of 1% per year. At the age of fifty, the rate jump to up to 3%, causing health issues:

- muscle stiffness
- aging joint
- wrinkles and fine lines
- lack of tone
- aging skin
- healing of wounds slower
- frequent fatigue.

Consuming more collagen will boost your body's collagen protection. So your daily collagen intake is recommended to represent 25 to 35% protein. The beneficial effects of an optimal collagen intake include intestinal health, less articular pain, less hair loss, better skin, and increased muscle mass.

## FOODS RICH IN COLLAGEN

Here are some of the best collagen-containing foods you can add to your diet:

**Bone broth**

Made by simmering bones, tendons, ligaments, and skin of beef, bone broth is an excellent source of collagen and several essential amino acids. It is also available as a food supplement.

**Spirulina**

This kind of seaweed offers an excellent source of plant-based amino acids.

**Codfish**

Codfish, like most other white fish, is a good source of collagen in addition to selenium, vitamin B6 and phosphorus.

**Eggs**

Eggs are a good source of collagen, including glycine and proline.

**Gelatin**

Gelatin is one of the best collagen-rich foods available. This is why it is advised to include it in your weight-loss diet.

# GOOD FATS AND BAD FATS

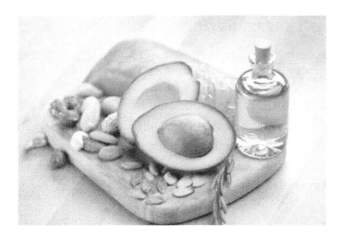

Fat is an essential macronutrient in food, so you must understand the following information to guide your diet journey.

## WHY IS FAT ESSENTIAL FOR YOUR HEALTH?

Dietary fats are found in both animals and vegetables and are essential for your living since they provide your body energy and support cell growth.

Fats also provide some valuable benefits and play essential roles, including:

- help your body absorb nutrients, including vitamins A, D, E, and K.
- help your body produce the necessary hormones.
- regulate inflammation and immunity issues.
- maintain the health of your body's cells (e.g., skin, hair cells)

## HOW MANY DIFFERENT FATS ARE THERE?

There are four major fats in food based on their chemical structures and physical properties:

• Saturated fat (bad fat) is a fat or lipid in which the fatty acid carbon chain holds maximum hydrogen atoms (i.e., saturated with hydrogens). This form of saturated fat is associated with various adverse health effects, while some recent studies moderate the popular belief and question how bad they impact health.

- trans fat (bad fat): (trans-unsaturated fatty acids or trans fatty acids) are a form of unsaturated fat associated with various negative health outcomes
- monounsaturated fats (healthy fat): are a type of unsaturated fat but have only one double bond. Adequate consumption of these fats is associated with positive health outcomes and may replace bad fats. Examples of monounsaturated fats sources include olive oil, avocados, and some nuts
- polyunsaturated fat (healthy fat) comprises two major classes, omega-3, and omega-6 fatty acids

## WHAT IS CHOLESTEROL?

Cholesterol is a fat present in all the cells in your body. Plus, your body needs some cholesterol to produce steroid hormones, vitamin D, and bile acid that helps you digest fats. Contrary to popular belief, your body makes almost all the cholesterol it needs in the liver. Cholesterol is supplied in small quantities (less than 15%) by plant and animal foods.

More than 85% of the cholesterol in your bloodstream comes from your liver rather than the food you eat. Dietary cholesterol has little impact on raising blood cholesterol levels, which is valuable information from a diet perspective.

While a high cholesterol level in the blood can be dangerous, maintaining the right cholesterol balance is essential for your health.

## WHAT TYPES OF FAT SHOULD YOU EAT?

It is recommended that you eat fats found naturally in food and not processed. Several healthy sources of fat exist, such as:

- Avocado (the fruit or avocado oil)
- Coconut (meat, cream, oil, milk, butter)
- Cacao butter
- Duck fat
- Medium-chained triglyceride (MCT) oil
- Pepperoni/salami/prosciutto
- Bacon fat/lard Beef
- Sardines, anchovies
- Salmon
- Olives and olive oil
- Macadamias and macadamia oil
- Almonds, Brazil nuts, hazelnuts, pecans
- Butter and ghee (to be consumed in moderation)
- Cream (to be consumed in moderation)

- Cheese (to be consumed in moderation)

## WHAT ARE FATTY ACIDS?

Fatty acids are a form of hydrocarbon chains with carboxyl at one end and methyl at the other. The biological activity of fatty acids is determined by the length of their carbon chain and their double bonds' number and position.

Saturated fatty acids and unsaturated fatty acids differ in their molecular structure. Unsaturated fatty acids are referred to as Dietary polyunsaturated fatty acids (PUFAs) and have been associated with cholesterol-lowering properties. The two families of PUFA are omega-3 and omega-6.

## WHAT ARE OMEGA-3 FATTY ACIDS?

Omega-3 fatty acids are polyunsaturated fats that the human body can't produce. Thus, you need to get these essential fats from your diet.

There are various types of omega-3 fats, which differ in their chemical structure. The three most common types of omega-3 are :

- eicosapentaenoic acid (EPA)
- docosahexaenoic acid (DHA)
- alpha-linolenic acid (ALA)

Omega-3 fats play a crucial role in your body:

- improves heart health
- supports mental health
- reduces weight and waist size
- decreases liver fat
- supports infant brain development
- fights inflammation

- prevents dementia
- promotes bone health

Omega-3 are essential fats that you must integrate into your healthy and balanced diet for diabetes. They have significant benefits for your heart, brain, and metabolism. However, recent studies have found that increasing your intake of omega-3 does not affect *blood glucose control*.

### WHAT ARE OMEGA-6 FATTY ACIDS?

Like omega-3, omega-6 fatty acids are polyunsaturated fatty acids.

Omega-6 fatty acids are primarily used for energy, so you need to get them from your diet in the right quantities.

Following different recommendations and guidelines, we recommend a ratio of 4/1 omega-6 to omega-3 or less, which means that for 400 milligrams of omega-6, you have to consume 100 milligrams of omega-3. However, the Western diet has a high ratio between 10/1 and 50/1.

### WHY AND HOW IS THE EXCESS OF OMEGA-6 HARMFUL?

A high amount of omega-6 polyunsaturated fatty acids associated with a very high ratio of omega-6/omega-3 is a constant in most Western diets, including the keto diet. That increases the pathogenesis of several diseases, such as cancer, cardiovascular disease, and autoimmune and inflammatory diseases. Conversely, high levels of omega-3 associated with a low ratio of omega-6/omega-3 induce health benefits. For example, a ratio of omega-6/omega-3 of 4/1 was correlated to a 70% reduction in mortality.

Consuming fatty fish twice a week, eating whole foods, and choosing dairy products and meat from grass-fed animals can help you improve your omega-6:omega-3 ratio.

# UNDERSTANDING THE ROLE OF MICRONUTRIENTS IN DIABETES MANAGEMENT

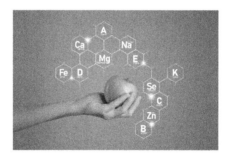

Micronutrients, often known as vitamins, minerals, and trace elements, are vital for overall health, well-being, and proper functioning of the body. Micronutrients do not provide energy and are active at very low doses. However, their importance is critical, and deficiency in any of them can have devastating health consequences.

Indeed, micronutrients are involved in all elementary metabolic reactions and play an essential role in metabolism and tissue function maintenance. Single micronutrient deficiency can easily be identified and treated. A poor single micronutrient status can be associated with the following various signs, including

- fatigue with difficulty in sleeping
- non-restorative sleep
- irritability
- intellectual impairments
- important stress
- paleness
- difficulty in digesting correctly
- repeated headaches
- permanent muscular tension
- palpitations

The most common single micronutrient deficiency are:

- **iron** deficiency
- **vitamin D** deficiency
- **iodine** deficiency
- **calcium** deficiency
- **vitamin B12 or B9** deficiency
- **vitamin A** deficiency
- **zinc** deficiency
- **magnesium** deficiency

## THE ROLE OF MICRONUTRIENTS IN MANAGING DIABETES

The use of micronutrient supplements in developed countries has increased substantially due to growing evidence that specific vitamins and minerals have beneficial roles in managing T2DM. Clinical solid evidence is emerging about the therapeutic benefits of vitamin D, vitamin K, and magnesium in improving blood sugar control and significantly reducing the risks of diabetes complications such as cardiovascular disease, stroke, kidney failure, diabetic retinopathy, and diabetic foot ulcers.

## VITAMIN D AND DIABETES COMPLICATIONS

Several epidemiological investigations have shown the protective effect of vitamin D against cardiovascular disease (CVD), one of the main complications of diabetes. In one study, a vitamin D [25(OH)D] level of fewer than 30 nanograms/mL (75 nmol/L) is linked with hypertension, diabetes, and hyperlipidemia in two-thirds of patients. This corresponds to an increased risk of developing heart disease compared with patients with vitamin D [25(OH)D] levels equal to and higher than 30 nanograms/mL (75 nmol/L).

Low vitamin D [25(OH)D] levels produce poor outcomes, particularly in individuals with diabetes. **Vitamin D deficiency —vitamin D [25(OH)D] lower than 30 nanograms/mL (75 nmol/L) was found to raise the risk of developing sudden cardiac death, heart failure, or incident hypertension significantly in people with diabetes.**

Vitamin D deficiency is associated with the following:

- increased microvascular complications (nephropathy, retinopathy, and neuropathy)
- increased cardiovascular disease
- increased diabetic retinopathy
- increased diabetic foot ulcers
- increased kidney diseases
- increased inflammation

---

## HOW CAN YOU GET ENOUGH VITAMIN D?

You can obtain the most vitamin D from the sun from about late March to the end of September. Your body produces vitamin D from direct sunlight radiation on the skin.

Food and dietary supplements are good sources of vitamin D, especially in the winter months. Vitamin D is generally found in oily fish (salmon, trout, mackerel, sardines, herring, and tuna), fish liver oil, and egg yolks. Vitamin D is also present naturally in low amounts in mushrooms exposed to the sun in the form of vitamin D2.

However, there are less than 120 IU in a cup of milk (250 mL) or vitamin D-fortified juice. Multivitamins are poor in vitamin D because the published RDAs are based on outdated and erroneous USDA recommendations. And taking several tablets won't solve the problem and may be harmful because of vitamin A toxicity.

**Here is a table of the Vitamin D Content of Selected Foods:**

- Cod liver oil: 34.0 mcg | 1,360 IU per 1 tablespoon. Be aware that just one tablespoon of cod liver oil can fulfill up to 250% of your daily vitamin A needs in one serving. And that prolonged daily intake of vitamin A may induce severe toxicity with various damages, including jaundice, liver injury, enlargement of the liver, and cirrhosis.
- Trout (rainbow), farmed, cooked: 16.2 mcg | 645 IU per 3 ounces
- Salmon, cooked, 3 ounces: 14.2 mcg | 570 IU per 3 ounces
- Swordfish (cooked). 3 ounces: 14.15 mcg | 566 IU
- Mushrooms, white, raw, sliced, exposed to UV light: 9.2 mcg | 366 IU per ½ cup
- Milk, 2% milk-fat, vitamin D fortified: 2.9 mcg | 120 IU per 1 cup
- Milk, fortified. 1 cup: 2.87-3.1 mcg | 115-124 IU.
- Soy, almond, and oat milk, vitamin D fortified, various brands: 2.5-3.6 mcg | 100-144 IU per 1 cup
- Ready-to-eat cereal, fortified with 10% of the daily value for vitamin D: 2.0 mcg | 80 IU per 1 serving
- Yogurt, fortified with 20% of the DV of vitamin D. 6 ounces: 2.0 mcg | 80 IU.
- Sardines (Atlantic), canned in oil, drained: 1.2 mcg | 46 IU per 2 sardines

- Egg, 1 large, scrambled: 1.1 mcg | 44 IU per 1 egg
- Egg yolk: 1 large egg: 1.0 mcg | 41 IU
- Liver, beef, braised: 1.0 mcg | 40 IU per 3 ounces
- Tuna fish (light), canned in water, drained: 1.0 mcg | 40 IU per 3 ounces
- Cheese, cheddar: 0.4 mcg | 17 IU per 1.5 ounce
- Mushrooms, portabella, raw, diced: 0.1 mcg | 4 IU per ½ cup
- Swiss cheese. 1 ounce: 0.15 mcg | 6 IU.
- Chicken breast, roasted: 0.1 mcg | 4 IU per 3 ounces

---

## VITAMIN K AND DIABETES

Vitamin K exerts beneficial anti-calcification, anticancer, bone-forming, and insulin-sensitizing actions.

A good vitamin K status is associated with a myriad of health benefits, including prevention and treatment of arterial calcifications, improvements in bone health, especially osteoporosis, **enhancement in insulin sensitivity, reduction of the risks of diabetes complications, and prevention of cardiovascular diseases.**

Recent studies have found that vitamin K is essential in improving **glucose metabolism, increasing** sensitivity, and improving other metabolic functions.

Vitamin K deficiency is also linked to an increased risk of diabetes complications such as heart disease and stroke.

## HOW CAN YOU GET ENOUGH VITAMIN K2?

Eating a balanced diet containing vitamin K2-rich foods will allow you to get sufficient amounts. Some good sources of vitamin K2 include:

- Natto | serving: 100 grams | Vitamin K2 content: 1104 mcg
- Kale, cooked | serving: 100 grams | Vitamin K2 content: 817 mcg
- Mustard Greens, cooked | serving: 100 grams | Vitamin K2 content: 593 mcg
- Collard Greens, cooked | serving: 100 grams | Vitamin K2 content: 407 mcg
- Swiss Chard | serving: 100 grams | Vitamin K2 content: 830 mcg
- Broccoli, cooked | serving: 100 grams | Vitamin K2 content: 141 mcg
- Egg Yolk | serving: 100 grams | magnesium content: 16 mg
- Hard cheeses | serving: 100 grams | Vitamin K2 content: 77 mg
- Beef Liver | serving: 100 grams | Vitamin K2 content: 106 mcg
- Pork Chops | serving: 100 grams | Vitamin K2 content: 70 mg
- Chicken | serving: 100 grams | Vitamin K2 content: 60 mcg
- Goose liver | serving: 100 grams | Vitamin K2 content: 369 mg
- Black Bean Natto | serving: 100 grams | Vitamin K2 content: 798 mcg
- Pepperoni | serving: 100 grams | Vitamin K2 content: 42 mcg
- Salami | serving: 1 cup | Vitamin K2 content: 24 mg
- Butter | serving: 100 grams | Vitamin K2 content: 21 mcg
- Chicken wings | serving: 100 grams | Vitamin K2 content: 25.3 mg

---

## MAGNESIUM AND DIABETES

Magnesium is an essential nutrient to the human body, playing an indispensable role in promoting and sustaining health and life. As a critical cofactor for activating a wide range of metabolic enzymes and cell transporters, magnesium is required for the good functioning of several hundred chemical reactions in the body.

Magnesium is also indispensable for activating vitamin D because the hydroxylation of vitamin D in the liver and the kidneys is mediated by enzymes that require magnesium.

Poor magnesium status may expose people to vitamin D deficiency even if they get adequate sun exposure or optimal vitamin D supplementation.

**Therefore, only the activated fraction could affect the human body** without a sufficient amount of magnesium. The remaining vitamin D will stay inactive and unable to deliver the expected health outcomes such as improved glycemic response control, increased insulin sensitivity, and reduced risk of diabetes complications. Magnesium also directly improves types 2 diabetes glycemic control and insulin sensitivity.

RECOMMENDED INTAKES

The Recommended Dietary Allowances (RDAs) for adults for magnesium in the United States are:

- for 19 to 30 years old males, the RDA is 400 mg daily
- for 19 to 30 years old females, the RDA is 310 mg daily
- for 19 to 30 years old pregnant females, the RDA is 350 mg daily
- for 19 to 30 years old lactating females, the RDA is 310 mg daily
- for 31+ old males, the RDA is 420 mg daily
- for 31+ years old females (including lactating women), the RDA is 320 mg daily
- for 31 to 50 years old pregnant females, the RDA is 360 mg daily

## HOW CAN YOU GET ENOUGH MAGNESIUM?

You can get enough magnesium from food. Some good sources of magnesium include:

- leafy greens | serving: 1 cup | magnesium content: 157 mg
- dark chocolate (70% cocoa)| serving: 28 grams | magnesium content: 61 mg
- pumpkin seeds | serving: 28 grams | magnesium content: 150 mg
- cooked black beans | serving: 1 cup | magnesium content: 120 mg
- chia seeds | serving: 30 grams | magnesium content: 111 mg
- soymilk | serving: 1 cup | magnesium content: 63 mg
- almonds | serving: 30 grams | magnesium content: 80 mg
- spinach, boiled | serving: ½ cup | magnesium content: 78 mg
- cashews | serving: 30 grams | magnesium content: 74 mg
- dry buckwheat | serving: 28 grams | magnesium content: 65 mg
- peanuts | serving: ¼ cup | magnesium content: 63 mg
- avocado | serving: One medium avocado | magnesium content: 58 mg
- brown rice cooked | serving: ½ cup | magnesium content: 42 mg
- milk | serving: 1 cup | magnesium content: 24 mg
- salmon | serving: Half a fillet (178 grams) | magnesium content: 24 mg
- banana | serving: one large banana | magnesium content: 40 mg

# PART III
# UNDERSTANDING THE GLYCEMIC LOAD DIET FOR DIABETES

# FOOD, WEIGHT LOSS AND DIABETES

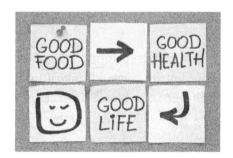

Eating to lower blood sugar spikes is not a one-size-fits-all approach. Different people, even twins, may respond to the same foods differently. However, following the glycemic load dietary pattern will ensure you get the most out of its beneficial effects. People who adhere to this diet more closely have consistently lower blood sugar levels, lower blood pressure, increased LDL cholesterol, reduced HDL cholesterol, and reduced triglycerides than those following other diets. It is considered healthier than modern fad diets (e.g., keto, low-carb, high-fat diets) because it is centered around eating low glycemic, whole, or minimally processed foods and avoiding high glycemic foods.

## DIET, WEIGHT LOSS, AND DIABETES

Hundreds of diets have been created with many promises regarding weight loss, inflammation reduction, and diabetes reversal. Low-carb and high-fat diets and low-fat diets were thought to be the best approaches to losing weight, controlling diabetes, and achieving a healthy weight. However, a growing body of evidence shows that these diets often don't work:

- low-fat diets tend to replace fat with easily digested carbohydrates.
- low-carb, high-fat diets overlook the importance of carbohydrates and often replace carbohydrates with highly processed fat-containing foods.
- fad diets often overlook the body's fundamental need for a balanced diet

The best diets that work restrict calories to some extent, supply sufficient and high-quality nutrients, avoid unhealthy foods, and balance hormones that help lower your blood sugar, improve your glycemic control, and regulate your weight. Diets do this in three main ways:

1. getting you to eat sufficient healthy foods and avoid bad ones
2. getting you aware of foods and nutrients you should include in your diet to achieve weight loss, better diabetes control, and prevent complications.
3. changing some of your bad eating habits and the ways you consider highly processed foods and refined carbohydrates

The best diet for losing weight and/or diabetes control is good for all body parts, from your brain to your heart to your pancreas. It is also a diet you can embrace and live with for a long time. In other words, a powerful diet rooted in nature that offers a flexible eating pattern provides healthy choices, banishes unhealthy foods, and doesn't require an extensive (and probably expensive) shopping list or supplements.

———

A healthy balanced diet with sufficient and adequate nutritional elements is critical for battling diabetes, weight gain, and obesity. Both nutritional deficiency and excess are tied to diseases and poor health conditions. Nutritional excess, particularly in highly-processed foods, refined carbohydrates, saturated fats, trans-fatty acids, sugar-sweetened foods, and sodium, can result in severe chronic inflammatory illnesses such as autoimmune disease, cardiovascular disease, bone disorders, diabetes as well as obesity. In contrast, nutritional deficiencies can lead to impairments of body function, fatigue, and conditions associated with vitamin and mineral deficiencies.

One diet that allows that is a Low glycemic load type diet. Such a diet —and its many variations—usually include:

- several servings of plant foods (e.g., vegetables, fruits) a day
- whole and minimally processed foods
- daily serving of seeds and nuts
- healthy fats and oils high in omega-3 fatty acids (canola, cod liver oil, fatty fish, flaxseed oil, Walnut oil, sunflower oil, etc.)
- lean protein mainly from fish, poultry, and nuts
- limited amounts of sodium
- minimal quantities of refined carbohydrates (e.g., white flour, white rice, white sugar, brown sugar, honey, corn syrup)
- limited alcoholic drinks
- NO high glycemic load foods
- NO trans fats
- NO highly processed foods

———

## DIETARY CARBOHYDRATES AND DIABETES

Increased carbohydrate-containing foods consumption with a higher glycemic index is found to cause a high spike in blood sugar and insulin release, making it harder to lose weight, control diabetes, and increase the risk of type 2 diabetes for healthy people. Conversely, eating carbohydrate-containing foods with a low glycemic load is associated with positive health outcomes and weight loss.

In addition, many studies have established that the quality of carbohydrates significantly impacts inflammation, weight gain, insulin resistance, and diabetes complications. Low-quality carbohydrates such as highly processed foods and refined carbs are associated with acute and chronic inflammation, impaired immune system responses, poor blood glucose control, and increased risk of diabetes complications. Conversely, high-quality foods such as whole foods or minimally processed food with low glycemic load are linked with lasting weight loss and better health outcomes, including improved control of blood glucose and reduced acute and chronic inflammation.

## DIETARY FATS AND DIABETES

Another essential nutrient you should consider as part of a glycemic load diet is fat. Eating enough good fat is necessary whether you are managing diabetes or aiming to achieve a healthy weight.

However, fats are higher in calories per gram than proteins or carbohydrates. A gram of dietary fat has nearly 9 calories, while a gram of carbohydrate has roughly 4 calories or protein has about 4 calories. Thus, you should be aware of serving sizes when eating fats.

Several studies have established that replacing trans fats and saturated fats with unsaturated fats (monounsaturated and polyunsaturated) reduces the risk of cardiovascular diseases in high-risk populations, including individuals with diabetes.

In addition, studies also found that replacing trans fats and saturated fat intake with low glycemic carbohydrates (e.g., whole grains, fiber-rich fruits, fiber-rich vegetables, and beans) results in cardiovascular benefits without altering blood glucose control.

On the other side, a growing body of evidence has revealed how dietary fat intake affects the inflammatory status and focused on the gut microbiome as an important factor explaining the increase of inflammation biomarkers and fat intake. Trans fats are tied with various adverse health effects, worsen inflammation, and trigger some diabetes complications. The consumption of high amounts of saturated fats increases the LDL cholesterol (bad form) and aggravates inflammation.

The American Diabetes Association recommends swapping saturated and trans fats in your diet with the healthiest alternatives, such as monounsaturated and polyunsaturated fats.

# THE GLYCEMIC LOAD DIET FOR DIABETES CONTROL AND WEIGHT LOSS

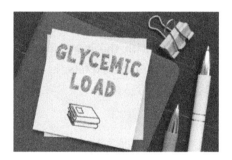

### THE GLYCEMIC INDEX DIET

The glycemic index concept was developed in the early 1980s to determine how carbohydrate-containing foods affect blood sugar levels scientifically. Since the initial research led by Dr. Jenkins took place more than 35 years ago, many scientists have identified that the glycemic index (GI) can be a powerful tool for maintaining weight, improving the effectiveness of weight-loss diets, and managing diabetes.

The glycemic index isn't formally a diet in the sense that you have to

conform to strict rules, follow particular meal plans or eliminate son.
foods from your daily meals. Instead, it's a scientific method of identifying how carbohydrates in foods affect blood sugar levels and
measuring how slowly or quickly they raise blood sugar. Thus, the
Glycemic Index referential is particularly important to know if you
want to maintain weight, lose weight, take more control of diabetes,
and fix some specific health issues.

The "glycemic index (GI) diet" refers to a targeted diet plan that uses
the glycemic index as the primary and only guides for meal planning.
Unlike other diet plans that provide a strict recommendation with a
specific ratio, the glycemic index diet (GI diet) doesn't specify the
optimal daily number of calories, carbohydrates, protein, or fats for
weight maintenance or weight loss. Instead, it provides an effective
eating plan with more flexibility and sustainable results in weight loss,
weight management, and diabetes control.

UNDERSTANDING GI VALUES

Glycemic index (GI) values are divided into three categories:

- low GI: This category comprises foods that have a GI value
  below 55
- medium GI: This category comprises foods that have a GI
  value in the range of 56 to 69
- high GI: In general, this category must be avoided because
  foods cause high spikes in the blood sugar level. Their GI
  values are equal to or higher to 70

Comparing the GI values may help guide your food choices. For
example, muesli has a GI value of approximately 86. A vegetable and
fruit smoothie drink has a GI value of 55.

ng to the Glycemic Index Diet looks simple because all know is where different foods fall on the 0 to 100 ˌex (GI).

• You fill up on low GI foods (GI value: 55 and under)

• Eat smaller amounts of medium GI foods (GI value:56 to 69)

• And mostly avoid high GI foods (GI value: 70 and up)

Besides referring to the glycemic index lists as needed, there is no complex weighing or measuring and no need to track your calorie intake. However, you will have to concoct your eating plan and menus yourself.

## HOW IS GLYCEMIC INDEX MEASURED?

Glycemic Index values of foods are measured using valid and proven scientific methods. GI values cannot be easily guessed just by looking at the composition of specific food or the nutrition facts on food packaging.

The GI measurement Follows the international standard method and provides commonly accepted values. (GI values can also be estimated with a good approximation through advanced data science tools.)

The Glycemic Index value of food is measured by feeding over ten healthy people a portion of the food object of the study and containing fifty grams of digestible carbohydrate and then measuring the effect for each participant on his blood glucose levels (blood glucose response) over the next two hours.

The second part of the process consists of giving the same partici-pants an equal carbohydrate portion of the glucose (used as the refer-ence food) and measuring their blood glucose response over the next two hours.

The Glycemic Index value for the food is then calculated for each participant by using a simple formula (dividing the blood glucose response for the food by their blood glucose response for the glucose (reference food)). The final value of the food's Glycemic Index is the average value for the participants (over 10).

Carbohydrates with a low GI value are more slowly digested, absorbed, and metabolized and induce a smaller rise in blood sugar and, therefore, usually, insulin levels.

Low glycemic diets or foods are associated with a reduced risk of chronic disease. Low glycemic index foods are known to release glucose in the blood slowly and regularly. Conversely, Foods that have a high glycemic index are known for their property of releasing glucose rapidly. Researches suggest that foods with a low glycemic index (LGI foods) are ideal for weight loss diets and foster lasting weight loss, in addition to their positive effect on the pancreas (insulin release), eyes, and kidney.

## The Glycemic Load Diet

The glycemic index provides a valuable tool to assess how carbohydrate-containing food affects your blood sugar. However, it doesn't inform you how high your blood glucose will go when you eat that food. The glycemic load was developed to provide a complete picture. It tells about how the food affects your blood sugar and how much pure glucose per serving it delivers.

Harvard researchers developed the glycemic load to provide a more helpful tool for tracking both carbohydrates' quality and quantity. The glycemic load of a specific food—computed as the product of that food's glycemic index value and its net carbohydrate content —has direct physiologic significance in that each unit of GL corresponds to the glycemic effect of ingesting 1 g of pure glucose. Typical low-glycemic diets contain from 50–150 GL units per day. For positive health outcomes, you are advised to maintain your daily glycemic load under 100. This will help keep your A1C level in the normal range and achieve a healthy weight if you are overweight or obese.

People with diabetes can eat up to 50 grams of sugar from all sources per day (in a 2,000-calorie diet). This means that you should target a GL of 50.

The Glycemic Load (GL) is computed using the following formula:

**Glycemic Load (GL) = GI x Net Carbohydrates (grams) content per portion ÷ 100**

Where net carbohydrate = total carbohydrates - dietary fiber

One unit of GL corresponds to the glycemic effect of ingesting 1 g of glucose. Typical low glycemic load diets contain 80–150 GL units per day.

Eating a portion of food with a GL of 10 is equivalent to ingesting 10 grams of glucose.

For example:

Let's consider a 1-cup serving size of quartered or chopped apple.

- net carb or available carbohydrate is equal to 14.3 grams.
- the glycemic index of an apple is equal to 38
- therefore the glycemic load is GL= 38 ÷ 100 x 14.3 = 5.4

**The glycemic load of a 1-cup serving size of quartered or chopped apple is equivalent to 5.4 grams of pure glucose.**

## THE GLYCEMIC LOAD RANGES

Like the glycemic index, the glycemic load (GL) of a food can be classified as:

- **low:** 10 or less
- **medium:** 11 – 19
- **high:** 20 or more

For a standard serving size of food, glycemic load (GL) is considered high with GL greater or equal to 20, medium with GL in the range of 11-19, and low with GL less or equal to 10. The Daily GL is the sum of the GL values for all foods consumed during the day.

As shown in the formula, the GL of a food is a product of 2 factors: the GI of the food and the net carb in food for a given serving size. And therefore, to increase or decrease GL, you must act primarily on the serving size. For example, medium-to-high GI foods like wheat bran bagels, barely bread, and watermelon have low GLs.

Eating many high-glycemic foods frequently increases the risk of diabetes complications, cardiovascular disease, and obesity. Conversely, eating low glycemic foods has been shown to help control type 2 diabetes, improve blood markers and improve weight loss.

Because there is a gap in the GL ranges, a food with a glycemic load (GL) of 10.1 is considered a medium GL. A food with a glycemic load (GL) of 19.1 is considered a High GL.

## THE GLYCEMIC LOAD OF A MIXED MEAL

Using GL values of individual foods to estimate the average GL value of a meal may be appropriate. You may add the GL values of foods to evaluate the glycemic load of a meal.

## FACTORS AFFECTING A FOOD'S GLYCEMIC LOAD

Many factors affect the glycemic load of food. These factors include:

**Food Processing Methods**: Food processing has been practiced for centuries in the form of cooking, dehydrating, fermenting, ultraviolet radiation, and salt preservation. However, modern food processing methods are more sophisticated and complex and alter foods considerably by adding many ingredients, including trans fats, high-fructose corn syrup, salts, artificial sweeteners, flavors, colors, and other chemical additives. The US Department of Agriculture (USDA) defines processed food as one that has undergone any procedure that alters it from its natural state. Highly Processed foods generally have a higher glycemic index and glycemic load because they contain added sugar and are so refined that you digest them more quickly than minimally processed alternatives.

**Ripeness**: when fruits or vegetables ripen, their nutritional compositions change significantly. Sugar content increases as the fruit or starchy vegetables mature as part of the ripening process. The starch in fruits or vegetables is transformed into sugars, and the proportion of simple sugar rises to roughly 20%. Therefore, ripe and over-ripe foods generally have a higher glycemic index and load than unripe foods.

**Physical form**: Complex carbohydrates are formed by sugar molecules linked together in complex and long chains. Complex carbohydrates are digested slowly and do not cause high spikes in your blood sugar. Conversely, the body quickly transforms simple or refined carbohydrates and induces powerful blood sugar spikes. Therefore, refined and simple carbohydrate-containing foods generally have a higher glycemic index and load than complex carbs.

## ■ SHOULD PEOPLE WITH DIABETES EAT A GLYCEMIC LOAD DIET?

Whereas the glycemic index is a good tool for making good food choices, the glycemic load goes beyond and helps to determine how different portion sizes of different foods compare. It allows you to eat the right serving sizes that would not cause high blood sugar spikes and would not release too much glucose into your bloodstream.

## WILL GLYCEMIC LOAD DIET HELP YOU LOSE WEIGHT?

Low-glycemic diets demonstrate much more short-term and mid-term weight loss than other diets. Eating low glycemic load foods and keeping your daily glycemic load under 100 is the key to weight loss and hormonal balance. A 2012-study published in "The American Medical Association" journal found low glycemic diets to be best and superior at maintaining weight loss compared to very low carbohydrate diets (like the ketogenic or keto diet) and low-fat diets. The findings support the low glycemic diet's assumption that "a calorie is not a calorie" and that "different kinds of food will affect us in different ways, despite having the same calorie number." Another 2014-study published in "The American Journal of Clinical Nutrition" supports low Glycemic and calorie-restricted diets as more effective than high Glycemic Index and low-fat diets for weight management and weight loss.

## LIMITATIONS OF THE CONCEPT

The glycemic index and glycemic load are great tools, but they do have a few limitations that you need to know:

- the lists of GI are quite limited. GI testing is new, and the process is expensive, time and resource-consuming.
- the glycemic index depends on some external intervention like cooking. Al Dente Pasta is known to have a Lower Glycemic Index
- the testing results may vary. As explained in the previous section, researchers rely on observing tests involving participants' metabolism to measure the glycemic index. This explains why GI may vary among studies.

Despite these limitations, the glycemic load diet provides powerful tools that will help you achieve your goals in terms of diabetes control, diabetes complications prevention, and weight loss.

# THE HEALTH BENEFITS OF THE GLYCEMIC LOAD DIET

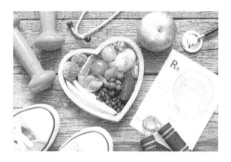

High insulin levels caused by high glycemic index foods are harmful and promote long-term high blood fat, high blood glucose, and high blood pressure and increase the risk of a heart attack. Because of this, following the glycemic load diet is beneficial in better managing diabetes, preventing diabetes complications, driving weight loss in the mid and long term, and improving your overall health.

Unlike other popular low-carbohydrate, high-protein diets, Eating a low Glycemic Load diet has been scientifically proven to help people, as you will see in this chapter:

- control blood sugar and insulin release
- achieve and maintain a healthy weight
- reduce PCOS symptoms
- maintain a healthy condition
- reduce the risk of type 2 diabetes
- improve women's gestational diabetes management and reduce adverse pregnancy outcomes.
- reduce the risk of developing metabolic syndrome dramatically
- prevent heart attack and stroke

## ◼ LOW-GLYCEMIC LOAD DIET AND INSULIN RESISTANCE REVERSAL

Insulin resistance is a serious and silent health condition that occurs when cells in your muscles, liver, and body fat start ignoring the signal that the insulin hormone is sending out to transfer sugar out of the bloodstream and put it into your body cells. As insulin resistance develops, the body reacts by producing more and more insulin to lower blood sugar.

Over time, the β cells in the pancreas working hard to make a higher supply of insulin can no longer provide more and more insulin. Your blood sugar may reflect the pancreas' inability to maintain the level in the healthy range, and your blood sugar rises, showing pre-diabetes or, at worst, type 2 diabetes.

Insulin resistance is silent and presents no symptoms in its first development stage. The symptoms appear later when the condition worsens, and the pancreas cannot produce enough insulin to keep your blood glucose within the normal range. When this occurs, the symptoms may be severe, including metabolic syndrome, polycystic ovary syndrome (PCOS), and various types of diabetes.

Fortunately, it is possible to reduce the insulin resistance effects and boost your insulin sensitivity by following a low-glycemic index diet.

Thus, for many of you, following a low-glycemic diet goes beyond weight-loss management and target the management of particular health condition sensitive to such kind of diet and particularly those related to insulin resistance like:

- excessive hunger
- lethargy or tiredness
- difficulty concentrating
- brain fog
- waist weight gain
- high blood pressure

## ◼ HIGH-GLYCEMIC INDEX FOODS AFFECT YOUR WEIGHT AND HEALTH.

Consuming high glycemic-load foods may be harmful to your health and causes weight gain because such foods will quickly raise your blood glucose level and cause a blood sugar spike compared to low glycemic foods.

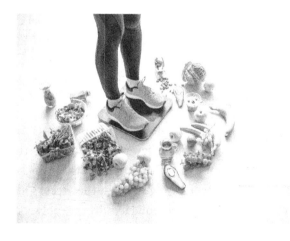

High-glycemic food consumption has also been associated with obesity, insulin resistance, fatty liver, metabolic syndrome, and a higher risk of chronic disease.

## ■ WEIGHT GAIN AND HIGH-GLYCEMIC INDEX FOODS

When you eat, food moves to your stomach and intestines, where it is broken down into macronutrients and micronutrients, which are absorbed and transported by your bloodstream. The pancreas produces insulin through its beta cells and releases it into the bloodstream when we eat to allow body cells, including muscles and other cells, to absorb and transform sugar (glucose) into energy throughout the body.

Insulin also sends signals to the liver, muscle, and adipocytes (fat cells) to store the excess glucose for further use:

- in muscle tissues as glycogen.
- in the liver as glycogen.
- in adipose tissue (fat reserves of the body) in the form of triglycerides.

## ■ LOW-GLYCEMIC LOAD DIET IS BETTER FOR YOUR BODY

Carbohydrates found in natural foods, such as legumes, fruits, vegetables, meats, fish, and grains, tend to be more complex and harder to digest, translating by a low-glycemic index. Eating such foods will lead to smooth increases and falls in your blood glucose levels, which help sustain your healthy condition, promote weight loss, prevent obesity, and helps diabetes control.

Many studies have also shown the health benefits of selecting foods with a low-glycemic index. Following a low glycemic diet may provide several health benefits, including:

- diabetes management (gestational diabetes, type 1 and type 2 diabetes)
- long-lasting weight loss,
- obesity control,
- reduction of heart strokes
- prevention of coronary heart disease
- PCOS prevention

## ■ LOW-GLYCEMIC DIET LOAD LEADS TO HUNGER-REDUCTION

Leptin, referred to as the starvation or "hunger hormone," is a hormone produced by fat tissues and is secreted into our bloodstream. It plays a crucial role in weight regulation by reducing a person's appetite.

Eating low-glycemic-index foods translates to eating a diet that lowers the insulin response and increases circulating leptin levels inducing a post-meal condition favorable for reduced food consumption due to a lower person's appetite. This may be very beneficial in such situations:

- type 2 diabetes management
- obesity control
- weight loss
- weight maintenance management
- insulin resistance

When you eat a good combination of foods, you will notice that your appetite is under control due to the leptin effect. Your insulin levels will also stabilize, and your sugar levels will rise and fall smoothly. The consequence will be beneficial since eating less often will lead to weight loss and a healthy lifestyle.

# CARB COUNTING VS. THE GLYCEMIC LOAD

*New studies suggest that the amount of carbs in a meal has a less significant impact on your blood glucose and insulin changes than the glycemic load. The glycemic load is a better predictor of blood sugar and insulin rise after a meal than carb count.*

---

## CARB COUNTING GUIDELINES FOR DIABETES

It is well established now that both the amount and the type of carbohydrates in food affect blood sugar levels. The total amount of carbohydrates in food was believed to predict the blood glucose response well. Thus, eating fifty grams of pure sugar would cause the same blood glucose response as any fifty-gram carbohydrate-containing food. Which is completely wrong!!!

Carbohydrates in the food you ingest will raise your blood glucose levels. How fast they raise your blood glucose depends on the quality of the carbs and what you eat with them. For example, sugar levels in fruit or vegetable juice induce a notable spike in blood sugar levels, while sugar in whole fruits or vegetables is digested more slowly. Carbohydrates-containing foods will be slowly digested if consumed with fat, fiber, or protein, thus inducing smoother increases in blood sugar levels.

Carb, or carbohydrate counting, means you keep track of the carbohydrates in all your meals, snacks, and drinks. Carb counting is an essential tool for people with diabetes that help them match their activity level and medicines to the food they eat. For many people with diabetes, carbs counting is used as the primary tool to manage their blood sugar efficiently, which can also help them:

- avoid high spikes in blood sugar levels
- stay healthy longer and reduce the severity of some diabetes complications
- improve their quality of life.
- prevent diabetes complications such as eye disorders, kidney disease, foot ulcers, heart disease, and stroke

If you take mealtime insulin, also known as fast-acting insulin, you'll have to count carbohydrates to match your insulin dose to your intake of carbs.

## TYPES OF CARBOHYDRATES IN YOUR DIET

When you eat carbs, your body digests and breaks them down into glucose, which is absorbed into the bloodstream. As the glucose level rises, the pancreas releases insulin, passing sugar in your blood to your body's cells for energy or storage. Dietary carbohydrates can be divided into two categories according to their chemical composition:

- complex carbohydrates are formed by sugar molecules linked together in complex and long chains. Complex carbs are found in vegetables, fruits, peas, beans, and whole grains.

- simple carbohydrates are transformed quickly by the body and induce an increased sugar blood level. They are found in high amounts in processed foods and refined sugars. Simple carbs foods are also deprived of essential nutrients and vitamins.

## CHOOSING THE BEST CARBOHYDRATE-CONTAINING FOODS

The carbohydrates quality you eat is crucial in adjusting the level of some hormones that influences diabetes, and inflammation or control weight gain, including insulin, cortisol, leptin, and peptide YY. For instance, frequently eating low-quality carbs (i.e., high glycemic foods) will lead to frequent blood sugar spikes, which will:

- let controlling your blood sugar levels hard,
- promote or worsen inflammation,
- cause weight gain, obesity,
- cause insulin resistance for healthy individuals
- dysregulate cortisol levels.

Conversely, the soluble and insoluble fibers in whole foods (low glycemic foods) are known to offset glucose conversion, prevent higher insulin supplies, and avoid irregular blood sugar variations that induce an excess of cortisol and insulin release.

## HOW MANY CARBS SHOULD I EAT?

Eating to lower the levels of blood sugar is not a one-size-fits-all approach. Different people, even twins, may respond to the same foods differently because everyone's body is different. The amount of carbohydrates you can eat while staying in your target blood glucose range depends on some factors, including age, weight, and activity level.

On average, people with diabetes should target to get nearly 45% of their calories from carbohydrates. Thus, if you consume about 1,900 calories daily to maintain a healthy weight, you have to aim to eat about 900-1000 calories from carbs. Considering that carbs provide four calories per gram, fat provides nine calories per gram, and protein provides four calories per gram, you have to eat 225-250 grams of carbs a day.

You should eat nearly the same carbs at each meal to maintain your blood sugar stable throughout the day.

## HOW MUCH GL SHOULD I EAT PER DAY?

The glycemic load of a specific food—computed as the product of that food's glycemic index value and net carbohydrate content —has a direct physiologic sense in that each unit of GL corresponds to the glycemic effect of ingesting 1 g of glucose. (please refer to chapter 10 for more details)

Typical low-glycemic diets contain from 80–150 GL units per day. For optimal health outcomes, it is highly recommended to keep your daily glycemic load (GL) under 100. This will help you achieve a healthy weight and maintain your A1C level in the normal range. However, if you have diabetes, according to the most recent recommendations, you can eat up to 10% of your daily energy intake in sugar which translates to 50 grams of sugar from all sources per day in a 2,000-calorie diet. This means that you should target a GL of 50.

## SHOULD YOU USE CARB COUNTING OR THE GLYCEMIC LOAD TO MANAGE MY DIABETES BETTER?

Carbohydrate counting is essential for diabetes management, especially if you take fast-acting insulin. You'll have to count the carbs you eat to match your insulin dose to your carbohydrate intake.

Because both the quality and quantity of carbohydrates affect your blood sugar, using the glycemic load will be beneficial. The glycemic load will provide the missing tool that will allow you to choose high-quality carbohydrate-containing food and achieve better diabetes management.

# PART IV
# ADHERING TO THE
# GLYCEMIC LOAD DIET RULES

# EATING WHOLE AND MINIMALLY PROCESSED FOODS

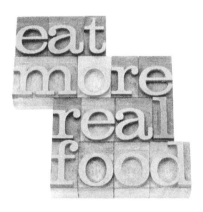

Highly-processed foods are generally industrially-made and contain many ingredients, including high-fructose corn syrup, trans fats, monosodium glutamate, artificial sweeteners, flavors, colors, and other chemical additives. They are believed to be a significant contributor to the obesity epidemic in the world, promoting diabetes, chronic inflammation, and the prevalence of autoimmune diseases. Therefore, you must identify healthy foods to include in your diet and those to exclude because they are considered unhealthy and pro-inflammatory.

Whole foods are unprocessed or minimally processed foods— nature-made foods without added sugars, fat, sodium, flavorings, or other artificial ingredients. They are generally close to their natural state, unprocessed, and unrefined. Whole foods have little to no additives or preservatives.

## A DIABETES-FRIENDLY DIET

**A diabetes-friendly diet** is a balanced, easy, long-term, and sustainable diet that selects low glycemic, whole, or minimally processed foods. It provides an eating plan centered around **unprocessed and minimally processed foods** and **excludes highly processed foods**.

This diet supplies your body with low glycemic, unprocessed, or minimally processed foods, with little to no unhealthy added constituents. You don't have to focus on calorie, protein, fat, or carb counting. Instead, you must concentrate on eating foods that do not cause high blood sugar spikes and release only reasonable amounts of glucose.

You can adopt a whole foods diet and still eat unhealthy carbohydrates-containing foods or fatty foods. Avoiding processed and refined foods is not the answer to better glycemic control, diabetes complications prevention, and inflammation reduction. Frequently eating carbohydrate-containing foods that cause high spikes in your blood sugar may make it difficult to control your blood sugar and put you at increased risk of diabetes complications.

Coconut, coconut oil, palm kernel oil, and palm oil fall in the category of whole foods or minimally processed foods but are full of saturated fats. Many experts, including the American Diabetes Association (ADA), and the American Heart Association, argue that replacing foods high in saturated fat with healthier alternatives may lower LDL cholesterol and triglycerides in the blood. In addition, oils rich in saturated fats are associated with increased inflammation and chronic diseases.

Thus the glycemic load component is critical to addressing such problems and providing a robust solution to achieve a healthy weight or win against diabetes.

# EATING LOW GLYCEMIC AND ANTI-INFLAMMATORY FOODS

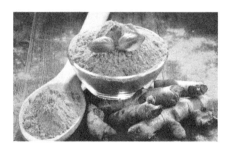

## EATING LOW GLYCEMIC LOAD VEGETABLES AND FRUITS

Vegetables and fruits constitute an essential part of a diabetes-friendly diet. A diet rich in low glycemic load vegetables and fruits positively affects your blood sugar and blood pressure. In addition, non-starchy vegetables and fruits are good sources of anti-inflammatory nutrients such as polyphenols, antioxidants, and flavonoids which contribute to lowering inflammation and, in turn, reducing the risk of diabetes complications.

The serving sizes for low glycemic load vegetables and fruits are equivalent to (please refer to part V for more details)

- 1 cup raw or salad vegetables
- ½ cup cooked vegetables
- ¾ cup (6oz) vegetable juice, homemade and unsweetened
- • ½ cup of cooked beans, lentils, and peas
- • 1 medium piece of fruit
- • 1 cup (6 oz) of sliced fruits
- • ½ cup (4 oz) of fruit juice

The total vegetable intake (per day) is equivalent to 8-10 servings. You have to vary your meals using the maximum recommended amount as follows:

• "Dark-Green Vegetables" group up to 2 servings

• "Red & Orange Vegetables" group up to 3 servings

• "Beans, Peas, Lentils" group up to 2 servings

• "Starchy Vegetables" group up to 1 serving

• "Other Vegetables" group up to 3 servings

The total fruit intake is equivalent to 2-4 servings per day.

---

## CHOOSING HEALTHY FATS

The glycemic load diet is rich in omega-3 and low in omega-6 than most diets. High levels of omega-3 combined with a low (omega-6/omega-3) are associated with many health benefits, including a significant reduction of unnecessary inflammation and diabetes complications. For example, a ratio (omega-6/omega-3) of 4/1 was correlated to a 70% reduction in mortality. So, based on recent studies, you have to keep the ratio (omega-6/omega-3) in the range of 1/1 and 4/1, which is associated with positive health outcomes.

Strategies to achieve an adequate ratio (omega-6/omega-3) include

meal without adding fats or salt. Therefore, you should consider integrating herbs into your daily diet when cooking.

Some strategies for getting more herbs and spices in your diet include

- using some fresh herbs as the main ingredient (e.g., herb salad, tabbouleh salad),
- replacing some green vegetables in salads with herbs,
- substituting (or reducing) salt in a recipe with spices,
- replacing mayonnaise with basil-olive oil preparation,
- drinking 3–4 cups of green tea daily.

---

## DRINKING MORE WATER

Water is critical for life. Without water, there is no life. All of the organs of our body, such as the heart, brain, lungs, and muscles, contain a significant quantity of water and need water to stay healthy.

Every day we lose water, and we need to replace it through a regular water supply. Otherwise, we can suffer from dehydration, which may alter the normal body's functions.

The recommended water intake for men aged 19+ is 3 liters (13 cups), and for women aged 19+ is 2.2 liters (9 cups) each day.

# AVOIDING HIGH GLYCEMIC AND INFLAMMATORY FOODS

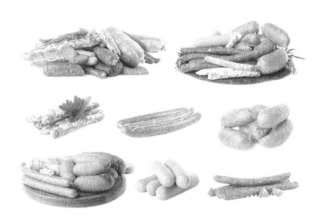

## LIMITING MODERATE GLYCEMIC INDEX FOODS AND AVOIDING HIGH GLYCEMIC FOODS

People living with diabetes must pay attention to the glycemic load of foods to prevent eating high amounts of glucose and experiencing abrupt spikes in blood sugar.

For a standard serving size of food, glycemic load (GL) is considered high with GL greater or equal to 20, medium with GL in the range of 11-19, and low with GL less or equal to 10.

You should then eat foods with GL under or equal to 10, and keep in mind that your daily allowance of GL must not exceed 50 (in a 2000-calorie diet)

---

## EXCLUDING TRANS-FATS CONTAINING FOODS

Trans-fatty acids are mostly industrially manufactured fats made during the hydrogenation process. Trans fats provide foods with a desirable taste and texture. However, unlike other dietary fats, consuming trans-fatty acids raises your bad cholesterol (LDL), lowers your good cholesterol (HDL) levels, increases your risk of developing severe cardiovascular conditions, and aggravates inflammation. Trans fats may be present in several food products, including:

- fried fast foods (i.e., french fries, fried chicken, battered fish, mozzarella sticks, and doughnuts)
- margarine
- peanut butter
- baked goods (i.e., cakes, cookies, and pies made with margarine or vegetable shortening)
- vegetable shortening

**Strategies to reduce drastically trans fats intake include**

- avoiding or reducing intake of fried fast foods—including french fries, fried chicken, battered fish, mozzarella sticks, and doughnuts, margarine, peanut butter, frozen pizza, baked goods made with margarine or vegetable shortening

- eating smaller portion sizes
- consuming trans-fat-containing foods less frequently.

---

## EATING A LITTLE LESS RED MEAT BUT ENOUGH PROTEINS

There is little evidence that red meat may contribute to inflammation and alter glycemic control. At the same time, some recent studies revealed that unprocessed red meats might be associated with less inflammation and are safe for people with diabetes or pre-diabetes. However, there is a consensus about the danger of consuming processed red meat such as sausage, bacon, salami, and hot dogs. A 2012 study funded and supported by some health and nutrition government agencies has established the link between processed red meal consumption and increased total mortality. It also revealed that daily unprocessed red meat consumption raised mortality risk by 13%. The study revealed that replacing one serving of red meat daily with other protein sources such as fish, poultry, and nuts could decrease mortality risk by 7-19%.

These findings suggest restricting your red meat intake reduces inflammation and prevents diabetes complications.

Eating adequate protein amounts is extremely important for your health because proteins play a crucial role in your body's vital processes and metabolisms. The weekly recommended proteins intake is equivalent to

- 30 servings of animal proteins (mainly lean white meat and eggs)
- 10 servings of seafood
- 5 servings of nuts and seeds

By restricting red meat intake in the range of 1/5 to 1/4 of animal proteins (e.g., 6 to 7.5 servings of red meat per week), you may experience improvement in your overall health and reduction of some symptoms caused by inflammation.

# PART V
# MANAGING DIABETES

# 5 STEPS TO MANAGE YOUR DIABETES FOR LIFE

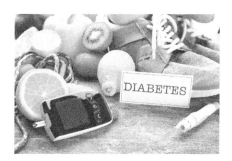

Unlike many health conditions, diabetes management outcomes depend mostly on you and require awareness and essential knowledge of what makes your blood glucose level rise and fall and how to manage these day-to-day elements. This involves adopting healthy eating to maintain your blood sugar under close control and prevent devastating complications.

You can manage your diabetes effectively and live a long and healthy life by following simple rules and caring for yourself daily. Diabetes, if poorly managed, can affect and harm almost every part of your body.

## 5 STEPS TO MANAGE YOUR DIABETES

Your plan for managing diabetes will help you better control your blood sugar and significantly reduce the risks of long-term complications. It includes the following steps:

### 1- MANAGE YOUR "ABC OF DIABETES."

And if indicated, stick strictly to the drug therapy prescribed by your doctor.

Managing your ABCs is one of the most critical steps in controlling diabetes. It shows how well your diabetes is controlled based on three measures:

1. hemoglobin **A**1C
2. **b**lood pressure
3. **c**holesterol (non-high-density lipoprotein [non-HDL])

(please refer to chapter 17)

### 2- FOLLOW YOUR DIABETES MEAL PLAN

The diabetes meal plan is based on the glycemic load diet for diabetes and the best and latest science. It will be your principal guide to getting healthy, balanced, and diabetes-friendly meals while controlling your blood sugar. It provides detailed guidelines for when, what, and how much to eat to achieve better diabetes management.

(please refer to chapter 20)

### 3- RECOGNIZE THE WARNING SIGNS OF HYPOGLYCEMIA

Hypoglycemia is common among people affected by type 2 diabetes who follow drug therapy and those affected by type 1 diabetes. You must act quickly to bring your blood sugar level back up when you have hypoglycemia. Severe hypoglycemia is a diabetic emergency when your blood sugar level drops so low. Therefore, you must recognize its warning signs and what to do to treat it promptly.

(please refer to chapter 19)

## 4- CREATE AND FOLLOW YOUR DIABETES DAILY ROUTINE

A diabetes daily routine is intended to create healthy habits that can lead to a better quality of life and prevent long-term complications. Your daily routine must include checking your feet to identify any injuries or changes to the skin or nails and **practicing regular physical activities** for at least 150 minutes per week (e.g., 30 minutes, 6 days a week).

## 5- STOP OR REDUCE SMOKING

Smoking makes managing diabetes challenging and regulating insulin levels difficult because active nicotine exposure may significantly lessen insulin action and decrease insulin release, causing smokers to need more insulin. Quitting smoking for good is associated with better glycemic control and reduced risk of diabetic complications.

# YOUR ABC OF DIABETES

Achieving hemoglobin **A**1C (<7%), **b**lood pressure (<140/90 mmHg), and **c**holesterol (non-high-density lipoprotein [non-HDL] <130 mg/dL) will significantly reduce the risk of devastating complications

---

If you have diabetes, three key steps—the ABC—can help you better control your diabetes and lower your risk of diabetes complications. The three steps are:

- A- Get a regular A1C (HbA1c) test to measure your average blood glucose and target to stay under 7% as much as possible.
- B- Try to keep your blood pressure below 130/80 mm Hg (or 140/90 mm Hg in some cases).
- C- Monitor your Total blood cholesterol, HDL cholesterol (good), LDL cholesterol (bad), and triglyceride levels with the help of your healthcare team.

## A- GET A REGULAR A1C (HBA1C) TEST

**Your diabetes is considered under good control if your A1c level is less than or equal to 7%. Beyond that value, the risk of developing diabetes complications increases.**

The A1C or HbA1c test is universally accepted as a reliable value of long-term glycemic control and a major driver of therapeutic decisions for patients with diabetes. The A1C test allows you to assess if your diabetes is under control.

A blood test is performed in a laboratory every three months to measure the hemoglobin level of red blood cells that have fixed glucose throughout their life. Your doctor will decide how often your A1C level has to be checked, but usually, you'll have to test twice a year. If your treatment is not meeting the therapeutical goals, you may need to get an A1C test more often.

The result of this test is important because it gives you a picture of your diabetes control during the past two to three months and indicates the risk of long-term complications.

Your diabetes is considered balanced if the A1c level is less than or equal to 7%. Beyond that value, the risk of developing diabetes complications increases.

**Increase in glycated hemoglobin**

Glycated hemoglobin (HbA1c) can be considered as evidence of your average blood glucose levels during the previous two to three months, as opposed to blood glucose which may fluctuate throughout time and provide information at a given moment. The higher the blood sugar level in the last three months, the higher the glycated hemoglobin value.

An elevated HbA1c level indicates an unbalanced diabetes control. Common causes of elevated HbA1c levels in people with diabetes include:

- an unbalanced and carbohydrate-rich diet
- insufficient dosage of anti-diabetic drugs or
- insufficient intake of insulin
- alcoholism
- gum disease
- anemia due to iron, folate, or vitamin B12 deficiency
- kidney disease and disorders
- high triglycerides
- thyroid disorders
- certain medications such as opioids, beta-blockers, some birth control pills, and statines
- excessive stress
- sleep disorder

## Reducing your HbA1c levels

Lowering HbA1c levels does not happen overnight but takes time. It is achieved by following a healthy diet and adopting a balanced lifestyle, such as the glycemic load lifestyle for people with diabetes. The 5-step plan will help you balance your diabetes, reduce your HbA1c level and avoid devastating complications.

---

## B- MANAGE YOUR BLOOD PRESSURE

**About two-thirds of adults with type 2 diabetes are affected by high blood pressure. You should keep your blood pressure below or equal to 130/80 mm Hg to prevent and delay some devastating diabetes complications.**

### What is high blood pressure?

Blood pressure varies throughout the day—from minutes to minutes and hour to hour based on your activities. It refers to the force exerted by the blood circulating against the walls of the body's arteries. Two numbers express blood pressure. The top number indicates the systolic or upper pressure and measures the arterial tension when your heart beats. The bottom number refers to the diastolic or lower pressure representing the vessels' pressure when your heart rests between beats.

Having blood pressure measures consistently > 130 mmHg for systolic and > 80 mmHg for diastolic results in the diagnosis of high blood pressure—hypertension.

The common risk factors include:

- unhealthy diets and eating habits—excessive salt consumption, high intake of saturated fat and trans fats, excessive coffee and tea consumption, low intake of fruits and vegetables
- bad lifestyle habits (poor physical activity, consumption of tobacco and alcohol)
- obesity
- family history of hypertension
- some medical conditions (e.g., diabetes or kidney disease)
- age over 65
- adverse effects of some medications

**Symptoms of High blood pressure**

Hypertension is usually silent and has no warning signs or symptoms —and most people do not know they have it. So, you must regularly measure your blood pressure to detect hypertension.

When symptoms begin, they may include

- headaches
- blurred vision
- nose bleeds
- irregular heart rhythms
- shortness of breath

- buzzing in the ears
- dizziness

Severe hypertension may cause:

- chest pain
- muscle tremors
- extreme fatigue,
- nausea and vomiting,
- confusion,
- anxiety.

**Medications for high blood pressure**

There are several medicines available for reducing blood pressure. Your doctor will offer you the appropriate medication. Drugs include:

- diuretics
- alpha-blockers and beta-blockers
- central agonists
- vasodilators
- calcium-channel blockers
- peripheral adrenergic inhibitor
- angiotensin receptor blockers
- angiotensin-converting enzyme inhibitors

**Complications of untreated hypertension**

Hypertension may cause severe damage to the heart, kidneys, brain, and other organs, including:

- heart attack
- strokes
- heart failure
- angina
- kidney failure

**Preventing and Treating High Blood Pressure**

Adhering to a healthy lifestyle is your first step to keeping your blood pressure in a normal range and lowering your risk of developing hypertension and its associated complications, such as heart disease and stroke. Practice the following healthy eating and living habits:

1. regularly monitor your blood pressure
2. take your hypertension medication (if applicable)
3. adhere to a healthy and balanced diet, such as the glycemic load diet
4. reduce your sodium intake
5. exercise regularly
6. achieve and maintain a healthy weight
7. stop smoking
8. drink alcohol in moderation

---

## C- CHOLESTEROL AND TRIGLYCIDES

Cholesterol is a lipid that is essential for life and made essentially by your body. Dietary cholesterol is exclusively present in animal foods such as meat, poultry, seafood, eggs, and dairy products.

Excess blood cholesterol or Hyperlipidemia is linked to an increased risk of heart disease and stroke because cholesterol deposits can build up in the walls of arteries that carry blood away from your heart to your body's tissues.

Cholesterol in your blood travels on proteins called lipoproteins:

- **low-density lipoprotein (LDL) cholesterol, referred to as "bad" cholesterol,** represents most of your body's cholesterol. Elevated LDL cholesterol level increases your risk for cardiovascular diseases.

- **high-density lipoprotein (HDL) cholesterol, referred to as "good" cholesterol,** absorbs cholesterol and returns it to the liver, which clears it from the body. High levels of HDL cholesterol can decrease your risk for cardiovascular diseases.

### Triglycerides

**Triglycerides are fat (also referred to as lipids) present in the blood, essential for life. When you eat, excess energy is converted into triglycerides and stored around the body,** commonly on your **hips** and **belly.** They are released in the bloodstream if your body needs energy more energy.

High triglyceride levels occur when you regularly eat more energy than you need.

A high triglyceride level added to high LDL cholesterol or low HDL cholesterol is linked with an elevated risk of cardiovascular diseases such as heart failure, heart attack, and stroke.

### Getting Your Cholesterol Checked

Monitor your Total blood cholesterol, HDL cholesterol (good), LDL cholesterol (bad), and triglyceride levels with the help of your health care team. (**Total cholesterol** is the global amount in your blood based on your HDL, LDL, and triglycerides numbers.)

# YOUR DIABETES MEAL PLAN

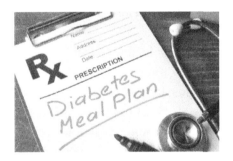

Adhering to the glycemic load meal planning for diabetes will ensure that optimal recommendations for a successful diabetes-friendly diet are met. Instead of giving strict recommendations, it gives you options for each food group you can choose. Each food proposed on the list has anti-inflammatory properties and a low glycemic load value.

All foods are also assumed to be:

- unprocessed or minimally processed
- in nutrient-dense forms

- lean or low-fat
- prepared and cooked with minimal added sugars, salt (sodium), refined carbohydrates, saturated fat, or trans fats.

An optimal daily intake of calories depends on your sex, age, and levels of physical activity, among other things. **You must eat a diabetes-friendly diet by following the general guidelines in part VI, "Meal Planning guidelines."** Recommended amounts of food in each food group are given to allow you to design your weekly and monthly eating plan.

You'll also have to:

1. **plan for regular, balanced meals** to prevent high or low blood glucose levels. Plan three meals daily with one or two low glycemic load snacks. This will help you keep your blood glucose under control.
2. **choose lower glycemic load foods and beverages** more often to maintain your blood sugar under control. choose when possible low glycemic load foods, and target to lower your daily GL (GL equal to 50 in a 2000-calorie diet)
3. **eat nearly the same amount of carbs** at each meal. Females with diabetes should target 45-60 grams of carbs per meal and 10-15 grams per snack. Males should target 60-75 grams of carbohydrates per meal and 15-20 grams per snack.
4. **use the plate method to plan your meals quickly.** The plate method is a visual way to ensure you get enough non-starchy vegetables and lean protein (low glycemic load foods) while limiting the amount of high glycemic load foods you eat. The plate composition is as follows: half is made up of non-starchy vegetables, a quarter is made up of lean protein, and one quarter is made up of low glycemic load complex carbohydrate-containing foods such as whole grains, starchy vegetables, or fruits.
5. **Stay hydrated.** Water is critical for life. Without water, there

is no life. Every day you lose water and need to replace it through a regular water supply. Otherwise, you can experience dehydration. Drinking enough water helps your body remove excess sugar through urine. **The recommended water intake for men aged 19+ is 3 liters (13 cups), and for women aged 19+ is 2.2 liters (9 cups) each day.** Contrarily, *low daily water intake is linked with an increased occurrence of dehydration and hyperglycemia.*

6. **choose healthy cooking methods**, such as broiling, roasting, stir-frying, or grilling.

7. **choose fresh or frozen unprocessed foods** or canned foods with no added salt or sugar.

8. **increase your olive oil consumption**. A minimum of extra virgin olive oil of four tablespoons per day is necessary to provide beneficial anti-inflammatory and antioxidant effects. When cooking, EVOO is an excellent choice as it has been well-established that it helps reduce blood pressure, lower bad cholesterol (LDL), and decrease inflammation.

9. **choose foods with no added sugar**. Added sugars aren't in foods naturally but are added. Examples of added sugars include glucose, fructose, dextrose, sucrose, lactose, high-fructose corn syrup, brown sugar, honey, cane juice, corn sweetener, and corn syrup.

10. **exclude Trans-Fats containing Foods.** Trans-fatty acids are mostly industrially manufactured fats produced during the hydrogenation process that adds hydrogen H2 to liquid vegetable oils to transform the liquid to a solid form at room temperature. Trans fats give foods an enhanced taste and texture. However, unlike other dietary fats, consuming trans-fatty acids raises your bad cholesterol (LDL), lowers your good cholesterol (HDL) levels, increases your risk of developing severe cardiovascular conditions, and certain cancers, and aggravates inflammation. Trans fats may be present in several food products, including fried fast foods, margarine, peanut butter, and vegetable shortening.

11. **Eat a little less red meat but enough proteins.** A 2012 study funded and supported by some health and nutrition government agencies has established the link between processed red meal consumption and increased total mortality. It also revealed that daily unprocessed red meat consumption raised the mortality risk by 13%. The study revealed that replacing one serving of red meat each day with other protein sources like fish, poultry, and nuts could decrease the mortality risk by 7-19%.

12. **avoid highly processed foods.** Ultra-processed or highly processed foods are defined as "formulations of several ingredients mostly of exclusive industrial use which, besides sugar, salt, oils, and fats, include food ingredients not used in culinary preparations, in particular, flavor enhancers, preservatives, colors, antioxidants, sweeteners, emulsifiers, and other additives used to provide sensory attributes of natural or minimally processed. Examples of ultra-processed foods include sugary drinks and fast foods, flavored potato chips, poultry nuggets and sticks, fish nuggets and sticks, powdered and packaged noodles, powdered and packaged instant soups, and powdered and packaged desserts.

# MANAGING LOW BLOOD SUGAR

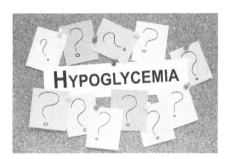

Blood glucose levels often change throughout the day. When they fall below 70 mg/dL, this is called hypoglycemia or low blood sugar. Hypoglycemia or hypo is common among people with type 2 diabetes —who follow a drug therapy such as insulin or other diabetes medicines—and people affected by type 1 diabetes.

You must act quickly to bring your blood sugar level back up when you have hypoglycemia. Severe hypoglycemia is a diabetic emergency when your blood sugar level drops so low. A person with a severely low blood level can't treat it himself and needs assistance.

If untreated, low blood levels can be dangerous. Therefore you need to know what causes it and what are its signs and symptoms.

**Symptoms**

Most people with diabetes experience hypoglycemia symptoms when their blood sugar drops to 70 mg/dL or lower. As undesirable as they may be, these symptoms are helpful as they let you know that your body needs a carbohydrate intake to correct low blood sugar. Common symptoms for Mild-to-Moderate include:

Fast or irregular heartbeat

- shaking
- abnormal sweating
- anxiety
- nervousness or Irritability
- dizziness and lightheadedness
- hunger

Symptoms of severe hypoglycemia include:

- loss of consciousness
- confusion and disorientation
- difficulty concentrating
- behavioral changes (e.g., Nervousness, Irritability, anxiety)
- convulsions or seizures
- coma

## WHAT CAUSES LOW BLOOD GLUCOSE IN PEOPLE AFFECTED BY DIABETES?

Many factors could lead to low blood sugar and include:

- taking too much insulin or medicines that help your pancreas release insulin into your blood.
- not eating or drinking enough carbohydrates. You risk

hypoglycemia if you don't eat enough carbs, delay meals, or skip meals while taking insulin or drugs, particularly sulfonylureas and meglitinides.

- fasting while taking insulin or drugs that lower your glucose level.
- too much exercise. Strength Training combined with low carbohydrate intake may cause insulin to drop quickly and cause hypoglycemia.
- hot and humid weather. People taking insulin or drugs that lower blood sugar have an increased risk of hypoglycemia because the body's metabolism is more effective in hot and humid weather, which leads to increased insulin absorption and efficacy.
- drinking alcohol. The biggest concern about drinking alcohol is hypoglycemia. With heavy alcohol consumption—while taking stronger medications such as insulin and sulfonylureas —the liver can not release enough glycogen to keep your blood sugar levels from dropping too low. Because it focuses on metabolizing the alcohol. This is especially true when you drink on an empty stomach.

## HYPOGLYCEMIA UNAWARENESS

Hypoglycemia unawareness happens when someone does not experience or notice the symptoms of hypoglycemia. If you have hypo unawareness, you need to check your blood sugar frequently to see if it is too low to correct it.

## HOW TO TREAT LOW BLOOD SUGAR?

If you think you have hypoglycemia, check it, or go ahead and treat it immediately because untreated hypoglycemia can be dangerous.

**The 15-15 Rule**

The 15-15 rule is used to treat hypoglycemia in the range of 55-69 mg/dL. It consists of increasing your blood glucose by ingesting 15 to 20 grams of fast-acting carbohydrates and checking your blood glucose after 15 minutes. If you're still below your target range, repeat these two steps until you reach your target range. Then eat a nourishing meal or snack to prevent your blood glucose from dropping too low.

15 to 20 grams of carbohydrate could be obtained from:

- 3 teaspoons of Sugar
- 3 Glucose tablets
- 3 teaspoons of Honey
- 3 teaspoons of corn syrup
- 1/2 cup (4 oz) of fruit juice or regular soda
- 1/2 cup (4 oz) of regular soda
- One slice of bread
- one small banana
- one medium apple
- 20 Grapes
- one regular yogurt
- 1/2 cup of Cooked pasta or couscous
- 1 cup of Milk (8 oz)

## TREATING SEVERE HYPOGLYCEMIA

Severe hypoglycemia is a dangerous condition that requires the intervention of your entourage. Therefore, they should be aware of how to recognize severe hypoglycemia and treat it. The treatment consists of giving you glucagon—the hormone made by the pancreas to raise blood sugar levels. Glucagon is only available with a prescription. It is administered to people with severe hypoglycemia and loss of consciousness. There are two types of glucagon: nasal and injectable.

You should ensure that some of the people around you are instructed on how to administer glucagon. You should also inform them where you stored it and when to use it.

# PART VI
# MEAL PLANNING GUIDELINES

# MEAL PLANNING GUIDELINES

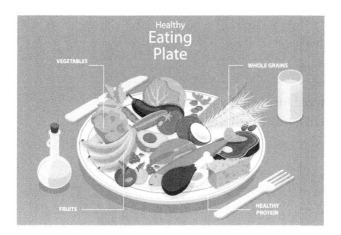

Meal planning allows you to make making informed choices that are diabetes-friendly and will work for your personal daily life and tastes. It will ensure that optimal recommendations for a successful diabetes-friendly diet are met. Instead of giving strict recommendations, it gives you options for each food group you can choose.

All foods are assumed to be:

- low glycemic load
- unprocessed or minimally processed
- in nutrient-dense forms
- lean or low-fat

prepared and cooked with minimal added sugars, salt (sodium), refined carbohydrates, saturated fat, or trans fats.

The total daily calories depend on your personal needs. You have to follow the general guidelines in the next chapters. Recommended amounts of food in each food group are given to allow you to design your weekly and monthly eating plan.

The five categories of foods are:

- vegetables
- fruits
- grains
- dairy and fortified soy alternatives
- protein foods

# VEGETABLES AND VEGETABLES PRODUCTS

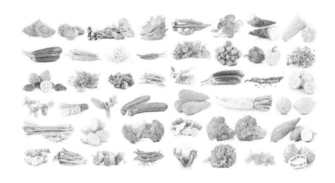

## WHAT IS THE PORTION SIZE?

The typical serving sizes for vegetables and vegetable juices are equivalent to:

- 1 cup raw or salad vegetables
- ½ cup cooked vegetables
- ¾ cup (6 oz) vegetable juice homemade and unsweetened
- ½ cup of cooked beans, lentils, and peas

All vegetables in this list are low-glycemic-index and anti-inflammatory

**How Much a Day?**

Total vegetable intake: up to 10 servings

- "Dark-Green Vegetables" group up to 2 servings
- "Red & Orange Vegetables" group up to 3 servings
- "Beans, Peas, Lentils" group up to 2 servings
- "Starchy Vegetables" group up to 3 servings
- "Other Vegetables" group up to 3 servings

---

For most people, following the low-glycemic diet will require an increase in total vegetable intake from all five vegetable subgroups ("Dark-Green Vegetables", "Red & Orange Vegetables", "Beans, Peas, Lentils", "Starchy Vegetables", "Other Vegetables").

**Strategies to increase total vegetable intake include**

1. increasing the vegetable content of mixed dishes (more vegetables)
2. adding vegetables to breakfast
3. blending and consuming vegetables into smoothies
4. preparing sauces with vegetables
5. consuming regularly vegetable-based soups

---

DARK-GREEN VEGETABLES: THE SIMPLIFIED LIST

- **amaranth leaves** (all fresh, frozen, cooked, or raw)
- **arugula (rocket)** (all fresh, frozen, cooked, or raw)

- **bok choy (Chinese chard)** (all fresh, frozen, cooked, or raw)
- **bitter melon leaves** (all fresh, frozen, cooked, or raw)
- **broccoli** (all fresh, frozen, cooked, or raw)
- **chamnamul** (all fresh, frozen, cooked, or raw)
- **chard (all fresh, frozen, cooked, or raw)**
- **collards** (all fresh, frozen, cooked, or raw)
- **dandelion greens** (all fresh, frozen, cooked, or raw)
- **endive** (all fresh, frozen, cooked, or raw)
- **escarole** (all fresh, frozen, cooked, or raw)
- **kale** (all fresh, frozen, cooked, or raw)
- **mixed greens** (all fresh, frozen, cooked, or raw)
- **mustard greens** (all fresh, frozen, cooked, or raw)
- **poke greens** (all fresh, frozen, cooked, or raw)
- **rapini** (all fresh, frozen, cooked, or raw)
- **romaine lettuce** (all fresh, frozen, cooked, or raw)
- **spinach (all fresh, frozen, cooked, or raw)**
- **swiss chard** (all fresh, frozen, cooked, or raw)
- **taro leaves (all fresh, frozen, cooked, or raw)**
- **turnip greens** (all fresh, frozen, cooked, or raw)
- **watercress** (all fresh, frozen, cooked, or raw)

---

## RED AND ORANGE VEGETABLES: THE SIMPLIFIED LIST

- **acorn squash** (all fresh, frozen, vegetables or juice, cooked or raw)
- **butternut squash** (all fresh, frozen, vegetables or juice, cooked or raw)
- **calabaza** (all fresh, frozen, vegetables or juice, cooked or raw)
- **carrots** (all fresh, frozen, vegetables or juice, cooked or raw)
- **red bell peppers** (all fresh, frozen, vegetables or juice, cooked or raw)

- **hubbard squash** (all fresh, frozen, vegetables or juice, cooked or raw)
- **orange bell peppers** (all fresh, frozen, vegetables or juice, cooked or raw)
- **sweet potatoes** (all fresh, frozen, vegetables or juice, cooked or raw)
- **tomatoes** (all fresh, frozen, vegetables or juice, cooked or raw)
- **pumpkin** (all fresh, frozen, vegetables or juice, cooked or raw)
- **winter squash** (all fresh, frozen, vegetables or juice, cooked or raw)

## BEANS, PEAS, LENTILS: THE SIMPLIFIED LIST

- **beans** (all cooked from dry)
- **peas** (all cooked from dry)
- **chickpeas (Garbanzo Beans)** (all cooked from dry)
- **lentils** (all cooked from dry)
- **black beans** (all cooked from dry)
- **black-eyed peas** (all cooked from dry)
- **Bayo beans** (all cooked from dry)
- **cannellini beans** (all cooked from dry)
- **great northern beans** (all cooked from dry)
- **edamame** (all cooked from dry)
- **kidney beans** (all cooked from dry)
- **lentils** (all cooked from dry)
- **lima beans** (all cooked from dry)
- **mung beans** (all cooked from dry)
- **pigeon peas** (all cooked from dry)
- **pinto beans** (all cooked from dry)
- **split peas** (all cooked from dry)

**Starchy Vegetables: The Simplified List**

- **breadfruit** (all fresh, or frozen)
- **burdock root** (all fresh, or frozen)
- **cassava** (all fresh, or frozen)
- **jicama** (all fresh, or frozen)
- **lotus root** (all fresh, or frozen)
- **plantains** (all fresh, or frozen)
- **salsify** (all fresh, or frozen)
- **taro root (dasheen or yautia)** (all fresh, or frozen)
- **water chestnuts** (all fresh, or frozen)
- **yam** (all fresh, or frozen)
- **yucca** (all fresh, or frozen)

---

## OTHER VEGETABLES: THE SIMPLIFIED LIST

- **asparagus** (all fresh, frozen, cooked, or raw)
- **avocado** (all fresh, frozen, cooked, or raw)
- **bamboo shoots** (all fresh, frozen, cooked, or raw)
- **beets** (all fresh, frozen, cooked, or raw)
- **bitter melon** (all fresh, frozen, cooked, or raw)
- **Brussels sprouts** (all fresh, frozen, cooked, or raw)
- **green cabbage** (all fresh, frozen, cooked, or raw)
- **savoy cabbage** (all fresh, frozen, cooked, or raw)
- **red cabbage** (all fresh, frozen, cooked, or raw)
- **cactus pads** (all fresh, frozen, cooked, or raw)
- **cauliflower** (all fresh, frozen, cooked, or raw)
- **celery** (all fresh, frozen, cooked, or raw)
- **chayote (mirliton)** (all fresh, frozen, cooked, or raw)
- **cucumber** (all fresh, frozen, cooked, or raw)
- **eggplant** (all fresh, frozen, cooked, or raw)
- **green beans** (all fresh, frozen, cooked, or raw)

- **kohlrabi** (all fresh, frozen, cooked, or raw)
- **luffa** (all fresh, frozen, cooked, or raw)
- **mushrooms** (all fresh, frozen, cooked, or raw)
- **okra** (all fresh, frozen, cooked, or raw)
- **onions** (all fresh, frozen, cooked, or raw)
- **radish** (all fresh, frozen, cooked, or raw)
- **rutabaga** (all fresh, frozen, cooked, or raw)
- **seaweed** (all fresh, frozen, cooked, or raw)
- **snow peas** (all fresh, frozen, cooked, or raw)
- **summer squash** (all fresh, frozen, cooked, or raw)
- **tomatillos** (all fresh, frozen, cooked, or raw)

# FRUITS AND FRUITS PRODUCTS

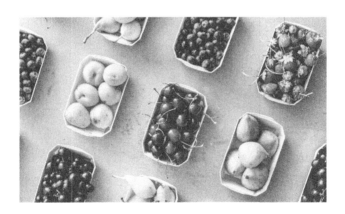

Having diabetes does not imply you can't eat fruit. Instead, you'll choose low glycemic load fruits. The majority of fruit and vegetables are nutrient-dense, low-calorie, and packed full of essential nutrients such as vitamins, minerals, and fiber.

## ◼ WHAT IS THE PORTION SIZE?

The typical serving sizes for fruits and fruits juices are equivalent to:

- 1 medium piece
- 1 cup (6 oz) of sliced fruits
- ¾ cup (6 oz) of fruit juice

All fruits in this list are low-glycemic-index and anti-inflammatory

**How Much a Day?**

2 to 4 servings per day

---

The fruit food group comprises whole fruits and fruit products (100% fruit juice). Whole fruits can be eaten in various forms, such as cut, cubed, sliced, or diced. At least 60% of the recommended amount of total fruit should come from whole fruit rather than 100% juice. Juices should be without added sugars or food additives.

For most people, following the low-glycemic diet will require increasing the total fruit. Strategies to increase total fruit intake include

1. often consuming fruits
2. adding fruits to breakfast.
3. choosing more whole fruits as snacks
4. blending and consuming fruits into smoothies
5. choosing and carrying fruit with you to eat later
6. creating adequate pairings with your favorite foods

---

■ FRUITS: THE SIMPLIFIED LIST

- **apples** (all fresh, frozen, dried fruits or 100% fruit juices)
- **Asian pears** (all fresh, frozen, dried fruits or 100% fruit juices)

- **bananas** (all fresh, frozen, dried fruits or 100% fruit juices)
- **blackberries** (all fresh, frozen, dried fruits or 100% fruit juices)
- **blueberries** (all fresh, frozen, dried fruits or 100% fruit juices)
- **currants** (all fresh, frozen, dried fruits or 100% fruit juices)
- **huckleberries** (all fresh, frozen, dried fruits or 100% fruit juices)
- **kiwifruit** (all fresh, frozen, dried fruits or 100% fruit juices)
- **mulberries** (all fresh, frozen, dried fruits or 100% fruit juices)
- **raspberries** (all fresh, frozen, dried fruits or 100% fruit juices)
- **strawberries** (all fresh, frozen, dried fruits or 100% fruit juices)
- **calamondin** (all fresh, frozen, dried fruits or 100% fruit juices)
- **grapefruit** (all fresh, frozen, dried fruits or 100% fruit juices)
- **lemons** (all fresh, frozen, dried fruits or 100% fruit juices)
- **limes** (all fresh, frozen, dried fruits or 100% fruit juices)
- **oranges** (all fresh, frozen, dried fruits or 100% fruit juices)
- **pomelos** (all fresh, frozen, dried fruits or 100% fruit juices)
- **cherries** (all fresh, frozen, dried fruits or 100% fruit juices)
- **dates** (all fresh, frozen, dried fruits or 100% fruit juices)
- **figs** (all fresh, frozen, dried fruits or 100% fruit juices)
- **grapes** (all fresh, frozen, dried fruits or 100% fruit juices)
- **guava** (all fresh, frozen, dried fruits or 100% fruit juices)
- **lychee** (all fresh, frozen, dried fruits or 100% fruit juices)
- **mangoes** (all fresh, frozen, dried fruits or 100% fruit juices)
- **nectarines** (all fresh, frozen, dried fruits or 100% fruit juices)
- **peaches** (all fresh, frozen, dried fruits or 100% fruit juices)
- **pears** (all fresh, frozen, dried fruits or 100% fruit juices)
- **plums** (all fresh, frozen, dried fruits or 100% fruit juices)
- **pomegranates** (all fresh, frozen, dried fruits or 100% fruit juices)
- **rhubarb** (all fresh, frozen, dried fruits or 100% fruit juices)
- **sapote** (all fresh, frozen, dried fruits or 100% fruit juices)
- **soursop** (all fresh, frozen, dried fruits or 100% fruit juices)

# GRAINS & BREAKFAST CEREALS

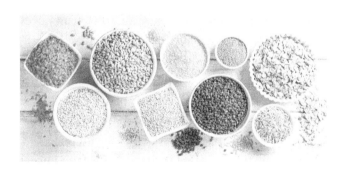

## WHAT IS THE PORTION SIZE?

The typical serving sizes for cereals and grains are equivalent to:

- ⅓ cup breakfast cereal or muesli
- ½ cup of cooked cereal, or other cooked grain
- ⅓ cup of cooked rice (white rice excluded), and other small grains
- ½ cup of cold cereal

All breakfast cereals in this list are low-glycemic-index and anti-inflammatory

**How Much a Day?**

Up to 3 servings per day.

---

WHOLE GRAINS: THE SIMPLIFIED LIST

- **barley** (all whole-grain products or used as ingredients)
- **brown rice** (all whole-grain products or used as ingredients)
- **buckwheat** (all whole-grain products or used as ingredients)
- **bulgur** (all whole-grain products or used as ingredients)
- **millet** (all whole-grain products or used as ingredients)
- **oats (Avena sativa L.)** (all whole-grain products or used as ingredients)
- **quinoa** (all whole-grain products or used as ingredients)
- **dark rye** (all whole-grain products or used as ingredients)
- **whole-wheat bread** (all whole-grain products or used as ingredients)
- **whole-wheat chapati** (all whole-grain products or used as ingredients)
- **whole-grain cereals** (all whole-grain products or used as ingredients)
- **wild rice** (all whole-grain products or used as ingredients)

# DAIRY AND FORTIFIED SOY ALTERNATIVES

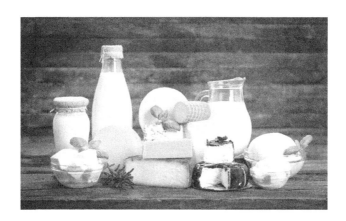

## WHAT IS THE PORTION SIZE?

The typical serving sizes for dairy products are equivalent to:

- 1 cup of milk, soy beverage, or yogurt
- ⅓ cup of cottage cheese
- 1 oz of cheese

All dairy and soy alternatives in this list are low-glycemic-index and anti-inflammatory.

People with celiac disease or lactose intolerance should consume dairy alternatives

**How Much a Day?**

Up to 3 servings per day

---

## DAIRY AND FORTIFIED SOY ALTERNATIVES: THE SIMPLIFIED LIST

- **buttermilk** (all fluid, evaporated milk, or dry including lactose-free and lactose-reduced products)
- **soy beverages** (all fluid, evaporated milk, or dry including lactose-free and lactose-reduced products)
- **soy milk** (all fluid, evaporated milk, or dry including lactose-free and lactose-reduced products)
- **yogurt** (without added sugar and food additives) (all fluid, evaporated milk, or dry including lactose-free and lactose-reduced products)
- **kefir** (without added sugar and food additives) (all fluid, evaporated milk, or dry including lactose-free and lactose-reduced products)
- **frozen yogurt** (without added sugar and food additives) (all fluid, evaporated milk, or dry including lactose-free and lactose-reduced products)
- **cheeses** (all fluid, evaporated milk, or dry including lactose-free and lactose-reduced products)

# PROTEIN FOODS

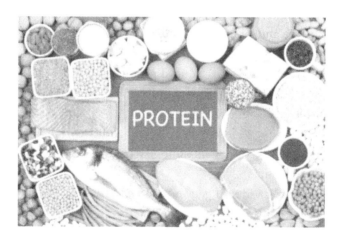

Eating a daily adequate amount of protein is very important for your health. Unlike carbohydrates and fat, your body does not store protein, and you need to eat enough to stay healthy. Animal-based foods are excellent protein sources because they offer a complete composition of essential amino acids with higher bioavailability and digestibility (>90%). Therefore, the main principle to observe here when designing your meal program is to keep a weekly proteins intake equivalent to:

- 30 servings of animal proteins (mainly lean white meat and eggs)
- 10 servings of seafood
- 5 servings of nuts and seeds

## MEATS, POULTRY, EGGS, SEAFOODS: WHAT IS THE PORTION SIZE?

The typical serving sizes for the "meats, poultry, eggs", "seafood", and "nuts, seeds, soy Products" groups are equivalent to:

- 3 to 4 ounces of cooked, baked, or broiled beef
- 3 to 4 ounces of cooked, baked, or broiled veal
- 3 to 4 ounces of cooked, baked, or broiled poultry
- 3 to 4 ounces of cooked or canned fish
- 3 to 4 ounces of seafood
- 2 medium eggs
- ⅓ cup of nuts (5 large or 10 small nuts)
- 2 tablespoons of nut butter
- 2 tablespoons of nut spread

---

## MEATS, POULTRY, EGGS: THE SIMPLIFIED LIST

Meats (lean or low-fats) include:

- beef, goat, lamb, and pork (fat red meats must be limited due to their pro-inflammatory effects). You have to choose lean meats preferably grass-fed beef, lamb, or bison
- game meat (e.g., bison, moose, elk, deer)

Poultry (lean or low-fats) includes

- chicken

- turkey
- cornish hens
- duck
- game birds (e.g., ostrich, pheasant, and quail)
- goose.

Eggs include

- chicken eggs
- turkey eggs
- duck eggs and other birds' eggs

---

## SEAFOOD: THE SIMPLIFIED LIST

Seafood include

- salmon
- sardine
- anchovy
- black sea bass
- catfish
- clams
- cod
- crab
- crawfish
- flounder
- haddock
- hake
- herring
- lobster
- mullet
- oyster
- perch

- pollock
- scallop
- shrimp
- sole
- squid
- tilapia
- freshwater trout
- tuna

---

## NUTS, SEEDS, SOY PRODUCTS: THE SIMPLIFIED LIST

Nuts (and nut butter) include

- almonds
- pecans
- Brazil nuts
- pistachios
- hazelnuts
- macadamias
- pine nuts
- walnuts
- cashew nuts

Seeds (and seed butter) include:

- pumpkin seeds
- psyllium seeds
- chia seeds.
- flax seeds
- sunflower seeds
- sesame seeds
- poppy seeds

# PART VII
# THE BEST FOODS (LOW GLYCEMIC LOAD FOODS)

# BAKED PRODUCTS

Apple Strudel ☛ Serving size= 1 oz, 28.4 g; GI= 59 (Medium); GL= 6.5 (Low); Net carb= 11 g

Bagel Multigrain ☛ Serving size= 1 miniature, 26 g; GI= 43 (Low); GL= 5 (Low); Net carb= 11.6 g

Bagel Multigrain With Raisins ☛ Serving size= 1 miniature, 26 g; GI= 49 (Low); GL= 6.1 (Low); Net carb= 12.4 g

Bagel Oat Bran ☛ Serving size= 1 miniature, 26 g; GI= 47 (Low); GL= 5.5 (Low); Net carb= 11.6 g

Bagel Pumpernickel ☛ Serving size= 1 miniature, 26 g; GI= 50 (Low); GL= 5.8 (Low); Net carb= 11.6 g

Bagel Wheat ☛ Serving size= 1 miniature, 26 g; GI= 71 (High); GL= 8.2 (Low); Net carb= 11.6 g

Bagel Wheat Bran ☛ Serving size= 1 miniature, 26 g; GI= 65 (Medium); GL= 7.5 (Low); Net carb= 11.6 g

Bagel Whole Grain White ☛ Serving size= 1 miniature, 26 g; GI= 72 (High); GL= 8.4 (Low); Net carb= 11.6 g

Bagel Whole Wheat ☞ Serving size= 1 miniature, 26 g; GI= 71 (High); GL= 8.2 (Low); Net carb= 11.6 g

Bagel, white ☞ Serving size= 1 miniature, 26 g; GI= 72 (High); GL= 9.5 (Low); Net carb= 13.2 g

Biscuit—Cheese ☞ Serving size= 1 biscuit (2 inch dia), 30 g; GI= 70 (High); GL= 9.8 (Low); Net carb= 14 g

Biscuit—Mixed Grain Refrigerated Dough ☞ Serving size= 1 oz, 28.4 g; GI= 70 (High); GL= 9.5 (Low); Net carb= 13.5 g

Biscuit—Plain Or Buttermilk Made From Recipe ☞ Serving size= 1 oz, 28.4 g; GI= 70 (High); GL= 8.5 (Low); Net carb= 12.2 g

Biscuit—Whole Wheat ☞ Serving size= 1 small (1-1/2 inch dia), 14 g; GI= 70 (High); GL= 3.9 (Low); Net carb= 5.5 g

Bread—100% Whole Grain ☞ Serving size= 1 slice, 1 oz, 28.4 g; GI= 53 (Low); GL= 5.9 (Low); Net carb= 11.2 g

Bread—Barley ☞ Serving size= 1 slice, 1 oz, 28.4 g; GI= 68 (Medium); GL= 8.5 (Low); Net carb= 12.5 g

Bread—Buckwheat ☞ Serving size= 1 slice, 1 oz, 28.4 g; GI= 47 (Low); GL= 6.2 (Low); Net carb= 13.2 g

Bread—Cinnamon ☞ Serving size= 1 slice, 1 oz, 28.4 g; GI= 72 (High); GL= 8.4 (Low); Net carb= 11.6 g

Bread—CornBread—Made From Recipe Made ☞ Serving size= 1 slice, 1 oz, 28.4 g; GI= 75 (High); GL= 9.3 (Low); Net carb= 12.4 g

Bread—Cracked-Wheat ☞ Serving size= 1 slice, 1 oz, 28.4 g; GI= 73 (High); GL= 9.1 (Low); Net carb= 12.5 g

Bread—Dough Fried ☞ Serving size= 1 slice or roll, 26 g; GI= 66 (Medium); GL= 7.5 (Low); Net carb= 11.3 g

Bread—Gluten-free multigrain ☞ Serving size= 1 slice, 1 oz, 28.4 g; GI= 73 (High); GL= 8.6 (Low); Net carb= 11.8 g

Bread—Italian ☛ Serving size= 1 oz, 28.4 g; GI= 70 (High); GL= 9.2 (Low); Net carb= 13.1 g

Bread—Italian Grecian Armenian ☛ Serving size= 1 small , 24 g; GI= 70 (High); GL= 7.9 (Low); Net carb= 11.3 g

Bread—Light Rye ☛ Serving size= 1 slice, 1 oz, 28.4 g; GI= 68 (Medium); GL= 6.5 (Low); Net carb= 9.5 g

Bread—Linseed Rye ☛ Serving size= 1 slice, 1 oz, 28.4 g; GI= 55 (Medium); GL= 4.7 (Low); Net carb= 8.5 g

Bread—Multigrain batch ☛ Serving size= 1 slice, 1 oz, 28.4 g; GI= 63 (Medium); GL= 7.5 (Low); Net carb= 11.9 g

Bread—Oat Bran 50% ☛ Serving size= 1 slice, 1 oz, 28.4 g; GI= 44 (Low); GL= 5 (Low); Net carb= 11.4 g

Bread—Oat Bran Bürgen ☛ Serving size= 1 slice, 1 oz, 28.4 g; GI= 49 (Low); GL= 4.8 (Low); Net carb= 9.8 g

Bread—Pita ☛ Serving size= 1 slice, 1 oz, 28.4 g; GI= 57 (Medium); GL= 8.7 (Low); Net carb= 15.2 g

Bread—Rice Bran ☛ Serving size= 1 oz, 28.4 g; GI= 66 (Medium); GL= 7.3 (Low); Net carb= 11 g

Bread—Rye ☛ Serving size= 1 slice, 1 oz, 28.4 g; GI= 59 (Medium); GL= 7.8 (Low); Net carb= 13.2 g

Bread—Soy ☛ Serving size= 1 oz, 28.4 g; GI= 44 (Low); GL= 4.7 (Low); Net carb= 10.7 g

Bread—Sunflower And Barley ☛ Serving size= 1 slice, 1 oz, 28.4 g; GI= 57 (Medium); GL= 5.2 (Low); Net carb= 9.2 g

Bread—Wholegrain pumpernickel ☛ Serving size= 1 slice, 1 oz, 28.4 g; GI= 46 (Low); GL= 3.3 (Low); Net carb= 7.2 g

Butter Croissants ☛ Serving size= 1 oz, 28.4 g; GI= 71 (High); GL= 8.7 (Low); Net carb= 12.3 g

Cake—Cherry Fudge With Chocolate Frosting ☞ Serving size= 1 oz, 28.4 g; GI= 55 (Medium); GL= 5.9 (Low); Net carb= 10.7 g

Cake—Sponge Made From Recipe ☞ Serving size= 1 oz, 28.4 g; GI= 55 (Medium); GL= 9 (Low); Net carb= 16.4 g

Churros ☞ Serving size= 1 churro, 26 g; GI= 66 (Medium); GL= 8.4 (Low); Net carb= 12.7 g

Coconut Custard Pie ☞ Serving size= 1 oz, 28.4 g; GI= 53 (Low); GL= 4.3 (Low); Net carb= 8.1 g

Coookie—Butter Or Sugar With Fruit And/or Nuts ☞ Serving size= 1 miniature/bite size, 5 g; GI= 69 (Medium); GL= 2.2 (Low); Net carb= 3.2 g

Corn Flour Patty Or Tart Fried ☞ Serving size= 1 patty, 10 g; GI= 75 (High); GL= 2.9 (Low); Net carb= 3.8 g

CornBread—Made From Home Recipe ☞ Serving size= 1 surface inch, 11 g; GI= 75 (High); GL= 3.4 (Low); Net carb= 4.5 g

Cornmeal—Fritter Puerto Rican Style ☞ Serving size= 1 fritter, 40 g; GI= 71 (High); GL= 5.6 (Low); Net carb= 7.9 g

Cornmeal—Stick Puerto Rican Style ☞ Serving size= 1 stick, 20 g; GI= 75 (High); GL= 6.9 (Low); Net carb= 9.2 g

Crackers—Cheese Regular ☞ Serving size= 1/2 oz, 14.2 g; GI= 67 (Medium); GL= 5.4 (Low); Net carb= 8.1 g

Crackers—Standard Snack-Type Sandwich with Peanut Butter ☞ Serving size= 1/2 oz, 14.2 g; GI= 69 (Medium); GL= 5.5 (Low); Net carb= 8 g

Crackers—Water Biscuits ☞ Serving size= 4 cracker 1 serving, 14 g; GI= 69 (Medium); GL= 6.3 (Low); Net carb= 9.2 g

Crackers—Wheat ☞ Serving size= 1/2 oz, 14.2 g; GI= 71 (High); GL= 6.1 (Low); Net carb= 8.6 g

Crackers—Whole-Wheat ☛ Serving size= 1/2 oz, 14.2 g; GI= 66 (Medium); GL= 5.5 (Low); Net carb= 8.3 g

Cream Puff Shell Made From Recipe ☛ Serving size= 1 oz, 28.4 g; GI= 55 (Medium); GL= 3.4 (Low); Net carb= 6.2 g

Croissant Chocolate ☛ Serving size= 1 oz, 28.4 g; GI= 73 (High); GL= 9.6 (Low); Net carb= 13.1 g

Croissant Fruit ☛ Serving size= 1 oz, 28.4 g; GI= 71 (High); GL= 8.9 (Low); Net carb= 12.5 g

Croissants Apple ☛ Serving size= 1 oz, 28.4 g; GI= 71 (High); GL= 7 (Low); Net carb= 9.8 g

Croutons Seasoned ☛ Serving size= 1/2 oz, 14.2 g; GI= 70 (High); GL= 5.8 (Low); Net carb= 8.3 g

Crumpet ☛ Serving size= 1 small, 20 g; GI= 73 (High); GL= 3.9 (Low); Net carb= 5.3 g

Danish Pastry—Cheese ☛ Serving size= 1 oz, 28.4 g; GI= 63 (Medium); GL= 6.5 (Low); Net carb= 10.3 g

Danish Pastry—Cinnamon ☛ Serving size= 1 oz, 28.4 g; GI= 63 (Medium); GL= 7.7 (Low); Net carb= 12.3 g

Danish Pastry—with Fruit (Apple, aspberry, Strawberry, Raisin, Lemon, Raisin) ☛ Serving size= 1 oz, 28.4 g; GI= 63 (Medium); GL= 8.2 (Low); Net carb= 13 g

Doughnut—Yeast-Leavened With Creme Filling ☛ Serving size= 1 oz, 28.4 g; GI= 55 (Medium); GL= 4.6 (Low); Net carb= 8.3 g

Doughnut—Yeast-Leavened With Jelly Filling ☛ Serving size= 1 oz, 28.4 g; GI= 55 (Medium); GL= 5.9 (Low); Net carb= 10.8 g

Dumpling Plain ☛ Serving size= 1 small, 18 g; GI= 63 (Medium); GL= 2.2 (Low); Net carb= 3.5 g

English Muffins 🐄 Serving size= 1 oz, 28.4 g; GI= 70 (High); GL= 8 (Low); Net carb= 11.4 g

English Muffins—Mixed-Grain 🐄 Serving size= 1 oz, 28.4 g; GI= 71 (High); GL= 8.8 (Low); Net carb= 12.4 g

English Muffins—Plain (Includes Sourdough) 🐄 Serving size= 1 oz, 28.4 g; GI= 73 (High); GL= 9 (Low); Net carb= 12.3 g

English Muffins—Whole-Wheat 🐄 Serving size= 1 oz, 28.4 g; GI= 70 (High); GL= 6.7 (Low); Net carb= 9.6 g

French Toast—Frozen—Ready-To-Heat 🐄 Serving size= 1 oz, 28.4 g; GI= 79 (High); GL= 7 (Low); Net carb= 8.8 g

Fritter Apple 🐄 Serving size= 1 fritter, 17 g; GI= 61 (Medium); GL= 3.5 (Low); Net carb= 5.7 g

Fritter Banana 🐄 Serving size= 1 fritter, 34 g; GI= 63 (Medium); GL= 6.9 (Low); Net carb= 11 g

Fritter Berry 🐄 Serving size= 1 fritter, 24 g; GI= 61 (Medium); GL= 4.3 (Low); Net carb= 7.1 g

Muffin—Cheese 🐄 Serving size= 1 muffin, 58 g; GI= 55 (Medium); GL= 9.4 (Low); Net carb= 17 g

Muffin—Whole Grain 🐄 Serving size= 1 miniature, 25 g; GI= 53 (Low); GL= 5.8 (Low); Net carb= 11 g

Muffin—Whole Wheat 🐄 Serving size= 1 miniature, 25 g; GI= 51 (Low); GL= 5.2 (Low); Net carb= 10.2 g

Pancake—Blueberry Made From Recipe 🐄 Serving size= 1 oz, 28.4 g; GI= 67 (Medium); GL= 5.5 (Low); Net carb= 8.2 g

Pancake—Buttermilk Made From Recipe 🐄 Serving size= 1 oz, 28.4 g; GI= 67 (Medium); GL= 5.5 (Low); Net carb= 8.2 g

Pancake—Plain Frozen—Ready-To-Heat (Includes Buttermilk) 🐄

Serving size= 1 oz, 28.4 g; GI= 72 (High); GL= 7.5 (Low); Net carb= 10.4 g

Pancake—Plain Frozen—Ready-To-Heat Microwave (Includes Buttermilk) ☛ Serving size= 1 oz, 28.4 g; GI= 75 (High); GL= 8.7 (Low); Net carb= 11.6 g

Pancake—Plain Made From Recipe ☛ Serving size= 1 oz, 28.4 g; GI= 67 (Medium); GL= 5.4 (Low); Net carb= 8 g

Pie Fried—Pies Cherry ☛ Serving size= 1 oz, 28.4 g; GI= 59 (Medium); GL= 6.7 (Low); Net carb= 11.4 g

Pie Fried—Pies Fruit ☛ Serving size= 1 oz, 28.4 g; GI= 59 (Medium); GL= 6.7 (Low); Net carb= 11.4 g

Pie Fried—Pies Lemon ☛ Serving size= 1 oz, 28.4 g; GI= 59 (Medium); GL= 6.7 (Low); Net carb= 11.4 g

Pie—Apple Made From Recipe ☛ Serving size= 1 oz, 28.4 g; GI= 59 (Medium); GL= 6.2 (Low); Net carb= 10.5 g

Pie—Blueberry Made From Recipe ☛ Serving size= 1 oz, 28.4 g; GI= 59 (Medium); GL= 5.6 (Low); Net carb= 9.5 g

Pie—Coconut Cream ☛ Serving size= 1 oz, 28.4 g; GI= 59 (Medium); GL= 4.7 (Low); Net carb= 8 g

Pie—Egg Custard ☛ Serving size= 1 oz, 28.4 g; GI= 59 (Medium); GL= 3.2 (Low); Net carb= 5.5 g

Pie—Lemon Meringue ☛ Serving size= 1 oz, 28.4 g; GI= 59 (Medium); GL= 7.7 (Low); Net carb= 13.1 g

Pie—Pecan Made From Recipe ☛ Serving size= 1 oz, 28.4 g; GI= 59 (Medium); GL= 8.7 (Low); Net carb= 14.8 g

Roll—Dinner Wheat ☛ Serving size= 1 roll (1 oz), 28 g; GI= 77 (High); GL= 9.1 (Low); Net carb= 11.8 g

Roll—Dinner Whole-Wheat ☛ Serving size= 1 roll (1 oz), 28 g; GI= 77 (High); GL= 9.4 (Low); Net carb= 12.2 g

Waffle—Plain Frozen—Ready-To-Heat ☛ Serving size= 1 oz, 28.4 g; GI= 75 (High); GL= 8.7 (Low); Net carb= 11.6 g

Waffle—Plain Made From Recipe ☛ Serving size= 1 oz, 28.4 g; GI= 69 (Medium); GL= 6.4 (Low); Net carb= 9.3 g

# BEEF, LAMP, VEAL, PORK & POULTRY

Beef-Offal—Heart: Braised, Broiled, Baked, Stewed or Fried ☛ Serving size= 3 oz, 85 g; GI= 0 (Low); GL= 0 (Low); Net carb= 0 g

Beef—Bottom Round: Braised, Broiled, Baked, Stewed or Fried ☛ Serving size= 3 oz, 85 g; GI= 0 (Low); GL= 0 (Low); Net carb= 0 g

Beef—Brain: Braised, Broiled, Baked, Stewed or Fried ☛ Serving size= 3 oz, 85 g; GI= 0 (Low); GL= 0 (Low); Net carb= 0 g

Beef—Brisket ☛ Serving size= 3 oz, 85 g; GI= 0 (Low); GL= 0 (Low); Net carb= 0 g

Beef—Brisket: Braised, Broiled, Baked, Stewed or Fried ☛ Serving size= 3 oz, 85 g; GI= 0 (Low); GL= 0 (Low); Net carb= 0 g

Beef—Chuck Roast: Braised, Broiled, Baked, Stewed or Fried ☛ Serving size= 3 oz, 85 g; GI= 0 (Low); GL= 0 (Low); Net carb= 0 g

Beef—Chuck Steak Varieties Chart ☛ Serving size= 3 oz, 85 g; GI= 0 (Low); GL= 0 (Low); Net carb= 0 g

Beef—Chuck Steak Varieties Chart: Braised, Broiled, Baked, Stewed or Fried ☛ Serving size= 3 oz, 85 g; GI= 0 (Low); GL= 0 (Low); Net carb= 0 g

Beef—Cuts of Steak: Braised, Broiled, Baked, Stewed or Fried ☛ Serving size= 3 oz, 85 g; GI= 0 (Low); GL= 0 (Low); Net carb= 0 g

Beef—Delmonico Steak: Braised, Broiled, Baked, Stewed or Fried ☛ Serving size= 3 oz, 85 g; GI= 0 (Low); GL= 0 (Low); Net carb= 0 g

Beef—Doner Kebab ☛ Serving size= 3 oz, 85 g; GI= 85 (High); GL= 6.4 (Low); Net carb= 7.5 g

Beef—frankfurter ☛ Serving size= 1 frankfurter, 45 g; GI= 28 (Low); GL= 0.5 (Low); Net carb= 1.8 g

Beef—Hanger Steak: Braised, Broiled, Baked, Stewed or Fried ☛ Serving size= 3 oz, 85 g; GI= 0 (Low); GL= 0 (Low); Net carb= 0 g

Beef—Kidney: Braised, Broiled, Baked, Stewed or Fried ☛ Serving size= 3 oz, 85 g; GI= 0 (Low); GL= 0 (Low); Net carb= 0 g

Beef—Liver: Braised, Broiled, Baked, Stewed or Fried ☛ Serving size= 3 oz, 85 g; GI= 50 (Low); GL= 2.1 (Low); Net carb= 4.1 g

Beef—Loin Steaks and/or Steak Types: Braised, Broiled, Baked, Stewed or Fried ☛ Serving size= 3 oz, 85 g; GI= 0 (Low); GL= 0 (Low); Net carb= 0 g

Beef—Mock Tender Petite Fillet: Braised, Broiled, Baked, Stewed or Fried ☛ Serving size= 3 oz, 85 g; GI= 0 (Low); GL= 0 (Low); Net carb= 0 g

Beef—Prime Rib: Braised, Broiled, Baked, Stewed or Fried ☛ Serving size= 3 oz, 85 g; GI= 0 (Low); GL= 0 (Low); Net carb= 0 g

Beef—Rib Steak Cuts: Braised, Broiled, Baked, Stewed or Fried ☛ Serving size= 3 oz, 85 g; GI= 0 (Low); GL= 0 (Low); Net carb= 0 g

Beef—Round Steak Varieties: Braised, Broiled, Baked, Stewed or Fried ☛ Serving size= 3 oz, 85 g; GI= 0 (Low); GL= 0 (Low); Net carb= 0 g

Beef—Short Loin: Braised, Broiled, Baked, Stewed or Fried ☞ Serving size= 3 oz, 85 g; GI= 0 (Low); GL= 0 (Low); Net carb= 0 g

Beef—Short Ribs: Braised, Broiled, Baked, Stewed or Fried ☞ Serving size= 3 oz, 85 g; GI= 0 (Low); GL= 0 (Low); Net carb= 0 g

Beef—T-Bone Steak: Braised, Broiled, Baked, Stewed or Fried ☞ Serving size= 3 oz, 85 g; GI= 0 (Low); GL= 0 (Low); Net carb= 0 g

Beef—Tenderloin: Braised, Broiled, Baked, Stewed or Fried ☞ Serving size= 3 oz, 85 g; GI= 0 (Low); GL= 0 (Low); Net carb= 0 g

Beef—Tongue: Braised, Broiled, Baked, Stewed or Fried ☞ Serving size= 3 oz, 85 g; GI= 0 (Low); GL= 0 (Low); Net carb= 0 g

Beef—Top Sirloin: Braised, Broiled, Baked, Stewed or Fried ☞ Serving size= 3 oz, 85 g; GI= 0 (Low); GL= 0 (Low); Net carb= 0 g

Beef—Tri-Tip: Braised, Broiled, Baked, Stewed or Fried ☞ Serving size= 3 oz, 85 g; GI= 0 (Low); GL= 0 (Low); Net carb= 0 g

Beef—Tripe: Braised, Broiled, Baked, Stewed or Fried ☞ Serving size= 3 oz, 85 g; GI= 0 (Low); GL= 0 (Low); Net carb= 0 g

Chicken—Backs and Necks: Braised, Broiled, Baked, Stewed or Fried ☞ Serving size= 3 oz, 85 g; GI= 0 (Low); GL= 0 (Low); Net carb= 0 g

Chicken—Breast Fillet Tenderloin: Braised, Broiled, Baked, Stewed or Fried ☞ Serving size= 3 oz, 85 g; GI= 0 (Low); GL= 0 (Low); Net carb= 0 g

Chicken—Drumstick: Braised, Broiled, Baked, Stewed or Fried ☞ Serving size= 3 oz, 85 g; GI= 0 (Low); GL= 0 (Low); Net carb= 0 g

Chicken—Leg: Braised, Broiled, Baked, Stewed or Fried ☞ Serving size= 3 oz, 85 g; GI= 0 (Low); GL= 0 (Low); Net carb= 0 g

Chicken—Tender: Braised, Broiled, Baked, Stewed or Fried ☞ Serving size= 3 oz, 85 g; GI= 0 (Low); GL= 0 (Low); Net carb= 0 g

Chicken—Thigh: Braised, Broiled, Baked, Stewed or Fried ☞ Serving size= 3 oz, 85 g; GI= 0 (Low); GL= 0 (Low); Net carb= 0 g

Chicken—Wing: Braised, Broiled, Baked, Stewed or Fried ☞ Serving size= 3 oz, 85 g; GI= 0 (Low); GL= 0 (Low); Net carb= 0 g

Eggs—Free-Range ☞ Serving size= 1 egg, 50 g; GI= (Low); GL= 0 (Low); Net carb= 0 g

Eggs—Free-Run ☞ Serving size= 1 egg, 50 g; GI= (Low); GL= 0 (Low); Net carb= 0 g

Eggs—Organic ☞ Serving size= 1 egg, 50 g; GI= (Low); GL= 0 (Low); Net carb= 0 g

Lamb—Breast: Braised, Broiled, Baked, Stewed or Fried ☞ Serving size= 3 oz, 85 g; GI= 0 (Low); GL= 0 (Low); Net carb= 0 g

Lamb—Cutlets: Braised, Broiled, Baked, Stewed or Fried ☞ Serving size= 3 oz, 85 g; GI= 0 (Low); GL= 0 (Low); Net carb= 0 g

Lamb—Leg: Braised, Broiled, Baked, Stewed or Fried ☞ Serving size= 3 oz, 85 g; GI= 0 (Low); GL= 0 (Low); Net carb= 0 g

Lamb—Loin: Braised, Broiled, Baked, Stewed or Fried ☞ Serving size= 3 oz, 85 g; GI= 0 (Low); GL= 0 (Low); Net carb= 0 g

Lamb—Neck: Braised, Broiled, Baked, Stewed or Fried ☞ Serving size= 3 oz, 85 g; GI= 0 (Low); GL= 0 (Low); Net carb= 0 g

Lamb—Rack: Braised, Broiled, Baked, Stewed or Fried ☞ Serving size= 3 oz, 85 g; GI= 0 (Low); GL= 0 (Low); Net carb= 0 g

Lamb—Rump: Braised, Broiled, Baked, Stewed or Fried ☞ Serving size= 3 oz, 85 g; GI= 0 (Low); GL= 0 (Low); Net carb= 0 g

Lamb—Shank: Braised, Broiled, Baked, Stewed or Fried ☞ Serving size= 3 oz, 85 g; GI= 0 (Low); GL= 0 (Low); Net carb= 0 g

Lamb—Shoulder: Braised, Broiled, Baked, Stewed or Fried ☞ Serving size= 3 oz, 85 g; GI= 0 (Low); GL= 0 (Low); Net carb= 0 g

Pork—back ribs: Braised, Broiled, Baked, Stewed or Fried ☞ Serving size= 3 oz, 85 g; GI= 0 (Low); GL= 0 (Low); Net carb= 0 g

Pork—Belly: Braised, Broiled, Baked, Stewed or Fried ☞ Serving size= 3 oz, 85 g; GI= 0 (Low); GL= 0 (Low); Net carb= 0 g

Pork—Cutlets: Braised, Broiled, Baked, Stewed or Fried ☞ Serving size= 3 oz, 85 g; GI= 0 (Low); GL= 0 (Low); Net carb= 0 g

Pork—Garlic Sausages: Braised, Broiled, Baked, Stewed or Fried ☞ Serving size= 3 oz, 85 g; GI= 0 (Low); GL= 0 (Low); Net carb= 0 g

Pork—Ham: Braised, Broiled, Baked, Stewed or Fried ☞ Serving size= 3 oz, 85 g; GI= 0 (Low); GL= 0 (Low); Net carb= 0 g

Pork—Loin: Braised, Broiled, Baked, Stewed or Fried ☞ Serving size= 3 oz, 85 g; GI= 0 (Low); GL= 0 (Low); Net carb= 0 g

Pork—Rib chops: Braised, Broiled, Baked, Stewed or Fried ☞ Serving size= 3 oz, 85 g; GI= 0 (Low); GL= 0 (Low); Net carb= 0 g

Pork—Roasts: Braised, Broiled, Baked, Stewed or Fried ☞ Serving size= 3 oz, 85 g; GI= 0 (Low); GL= 0 (Low); Net carb= 0 g

Pork—Sausages: Braised, Broiled, Baked, Stewed or Fried ☞ Serving size= 3 oz, 85 g; GI= 0 (Low); GL= 0 (Low); Net carb= 0 g

Pork—Shoulder chops: Braised, Broiled, Baked, Stewed or Fried ☞ Serving size= 3 oz, 85 g; GI= 0 (Low); GL= 0 (Low); Net carb= 0 g

Pork—Sirloin chops: Braised, Broiled, Baked, Stewed or Fried ☞ Serving size= 3 oz, 85 g; GI= 0 (Low); GL= 0 (Low); Net carb= 0 g

Pork—spare ribs: Braised, Broiled, Baked, Stewed or Fried ☞ Serving size= 3 oz, 85 g; GI= 0 (Low); GL= 0 (Low); Net carb= 0 g

Turkey—Backs and Necks: Braised, Broiled, Baked, Stewed or Fried ☞ Serving size= 3 oz, 85 g; GI= 0 (Low); GL= 0 (Low); Net carb= 0 g

Turkey—Breast Fillet Tenderloin: Braised, Broiled, Baked, Stewed or

Fried ☞ Serving size= 3 oz, 85 g; GI= 0 (Low); GL= 0 (Low); Net carb= 0 g

Turkey—Breast: Braised, Broiled, Baked, Stewed or Fried ☞ Serving size= 3 oz, 85 g; GI= 0 (Low); GL= 0 (Low); Net carb= 0 g

Turkey—Drumstick: Braised, Broiled, Baked, Stewed or Fried ☞ Serving size= 3 oz, 85 g; GI= 0 (Low); GL= 0 (Low); Net carb= 0 g

Turkey—Leg: Braised, Broiled, Baked, Stewed or Fried ☞ Serving size= 3 oz, 85 g; GI= 0 (Low); GL= 0 (Low); Net carb= 0 g

Turkey—Tender: Braised, Broiled, Baked, Stewed or Fried ☞ Serving size= 3 oz, 85 g; GI= 0 (Low); GL= 0 (Low); Net carb= 0 g

Turkey—Thigh: Braised, Broiled, Baked, Stewed or Fried ☞ Serving size= 3 oz, 85 g; GI= 0 (Low); GL= 0 (Low); Net carb= 0 g

Turkey—Wing: Braised, Broiled, Baked, Stewed or Fried ☞ Serving size= 3 oz, 85 g; GI= 0 (Low); GL= 0 (Low); Net carb= 0 g

Veal-Offal—Heart: Braised, Broiled, Baked, Stewed or Fried ☞ Serving size= 3 oz, 85 g; GI= 0 (Low); GL= 0 (Low); Net carb= 0 g

Veal—Bottom Round: Braised, Broiled, Baked, Stewed or Fried ☞ Serving size= 3 oz, 85 g; GI= 0 (Low); GL= 0 (Low); Net carb= 0 g

Veal—Brain: Braised, Broiled, Baked, Stewed or Fried ☞ Serving size= 3 oz, 85 g; GI= 0 (Low); GL= 0 (Low); Net carb= 0 g

Veal—Brisket: Braised, Broiled, Baked, Stewed or Fried ☞ Serving size= 3 oz, 85 g; GI= 0 (Low); GL= 0 (Low); Net carb= 0 g

Veal—Chuck Roast: Braised, Broiled, Baked, Stewed or Fried ☞ Serving size= 3 oz, 85 g; GI= 0 (Low); GL= 0 (Low); Net carb= 0 g

Veal—Chuck Steak Varieties Chart: Braised, Broiled, Baked, Stewed or Fried ☞ Serving size= 3 oz, 85 g; GI= 0 (Low); GL= 0 (Low); Net carb= 0 g

Veal—Cuts of Steak: Braised, Broiled, Baked, Stewed or Fried ☛ Serving size= 3 oz, 85 g; GI= 0 (Low); GL= 0 (Low); Net carb= 0 g

Veal—Delmonico Steak: Braised, Broiled, Baked, Stewed or Fried ☛ Serving size= 3 oz, 85 g; GI= 0 (Low); GL= 0 (Low); Net carb= 0 g

Veal—Hanger Steak: Braised, Broiled, Baked, Stewed or Fried ☛ Serving size= 3 oz, 85 g; GI= 0 (Low); GL= 0 (Low); Net carb= 0 g

Veal—Kidney: Braised, Broiled, Baked, Stewed or Fried ☛ Serving size= 3 oz, 85 g; GI= 0 (Low); GL= 0 (Low); Net carb= 0 g

Veal—Liver: Braised, Broiled, Baked, Stewed or Fried ☛ Serving size= 1 slice, 81 g; GI= 50 (Low); GL= 2.1 (Low); Net carb= 4.1 g

Veal—Loin Steaks and/or Steak Types: Braised, Broiled, Baked, Stewed or Fried ☛ Serving size= 3 oz, 85 g; GI= 0 (Low); GL= 0 (Low); Net carb= 0 g

Veal—Mock Tender Petite Fillet: Braised, Broiled, Baked, Stewed or Fried ☛ Serving size= 3 oz, 85 g; GI= 0 (Low); GL= 0 (Low); Net carb= 0 g

Veal—Prime Rib: Braised, Broiled, Baked, Stewed or Fried ☛ Serving size= 3 oz, 85 g; GI= 0 (Low); GL= 0 (Low); Net carb= 0 g

Veal—Rib Steak Cuts: Braised, Broiled, Baked, Stewed or Fried ☛ Serving size= 3 oz, 85 g; GI= 0 (Low); GL= 0 (Low); Net carb= 0 g

Veal—Round Steak Varieties: Braised, Broiled, Baked, Stewed or Fried ☛ Serving size= 3 oz, 85 g; GI= 0 (Low); GL= 0 (Low); Net carb= 0 g

Veal—Short Loin: Braised, Broiled, Baked, Stewed or Fried ☛ Serving size= 3 oz, 85 g; GI= 0 (Low); GL= 0 (Low); Net carb= 0 g

Veal—Short Ribs: Braised, Broiled, Baked, Stewed or Fried ☛ Serving size= 3 oz, 85 g; GI= 0 (Low); GL= 0 (Low); Net carb= 0 g

Veal—T-Bone Steak: Braised, Broiled, Baked, Stewed or Fried ☛ Serving size= 3 oz, 85 g; GI= 0 (Low); GL= 0 (Low); Net carb= 0 g

Veal—Tenderloin: Braised, Broiled, Baked, Stewed or Fried ☛ Serving size= 3 oz, 85 g; GI= 0 (Low); GL= 0 (Low); Net carb= 0 g

Veal—Tongue: Braised, Broiled, Baked, Stewed or Fried ☛ Serving size= 3 oz, 85 g; GI= 0 (Low); GL= 0 (Low); Net carb= 0 g

Veal—Top Sirloin: Braised, Broiled, Baked, Stewed or Fried ☛ Serving size= 3 oz, 85 g; GI= 0 (Low); GL= 0 (Low); Net carb= 0 g

Veal—Tri-Tip: Braised, Broiled, Baked, Stewed or Fried ☛ Serving size= 3 oz, 85 g; GI= 0 (Low); GL= 0 (Low); Net carb= 0 g

Veal—Tripe: Braised, Broiled, Baked, Stewed or Fried ☛ Serving size= 3 oz, 85 g; GI= 0 (Low); GL= 0 (Low); Net carb= 0 g

# BEVERAGES

**— People with diabetes must avoid heavy drinking**

Acai Berry Drink ☛ Serving size= 4 fl oz, 133 g; GI= 27 (Low); GL= 4.2 (Low); Net carb= 15.5 g

100 Proof Liquor ☛ Serving size= 1 fl oz, 27.8 g; GI= 0 (Low); GL= 0 (Low); Net carb= 0 g

86 Proof Liquor ☛ Serving size= 1 fl oz, 27.8 g; GI= 0 (Low); GL= 0 (Low); Net carb= 0 g

90 Proof Liquor ☛ Serving size= 1 fl oz, 27.8 g; GI= 0 (Low); GL= 0 (Low); Net carb= 0 g

94 Proof Liquor ☛ Serving size= 1 fl oz, 27.8 g; GI= 0 (Low); GL= 0 (Low); Net carb= 0 g

Beer ☛ Serving size= 8 fl oz, 266 g; GI= 100 (High); GL= 9.4 (Low); Net carb= 9.4 g

Creme De Menthe 72 Proof ☛ Serving size= 1 fl oz, 33.6 g; GI= 63 (Medium); GL= 8.8 (Low); Net carb= 14 g

Gin ☛ Serving size= 1 fl oz, 27.8 g; GI= 0 (Low); GL= 0 (Low); Net carb= 0 g

Liqueur Coffee 63 Proof ☛ Serving size= 1 fl oz, 34.8 g; GI= 63 (Medium); GL= 7.1 (Low); Net carb= 11.2 g

Muscat Wine ☛ Serving size= 4 fl oz, 133 g; GI= 7 (Low); GL= 0.5 (Low); Net carb= 7 g

Red Wine ☛ Serving size= 4 fl oz, 133 g; GI= 7 (Low); GL= 0.2 (Low); Net carb= 3.5 g

Rose Wine ☛ Serving size= 4 fl oz, 133 g; GI= 7 (Low); GL= 0.4 (Low); Net carb= 5.1 g

Rum ☛ Serving size= 1 fl oz, 27.8 g; GI= 0 (Low); GL= 0 (Low); Net carb= 0 g

Sauvignon Blanc ☛ Serving size= 4 fl oz, 133 g; GI= 7 (Low); GL= 0.2 (Low); Net carb= 2.7 g

Semillon ☛ Serving size= 4 fl oz, 133 g; GI= 7 (Low); GL= 0.3 (Low); Net carb= 4.1 g

Vodka ☛ Serving size= 1 fl oz, 27.8 g; GI= 0 (Low); GL= 0 (Low); Net carb= 0 g

Whiskey ☛ Serving size= 1 fl oz, 27.8 g; GI= 0 (Low); GL= 0 (Low); Net carb= 0 g

Whiskey Sour ☛ Serving size= 1 fl oz, 30.4 g; GI= 73 (High); GL= 2.9 (Low); Net carb= 4 g

White Wine ☛ Serving size= 1 fl oz, 29.4 g; GI= 7 (Low); GL= 0.1 (Low); Net carb= 0.8 g

Aloe Vera Juice Drink ☛ Serving size= 8 fl oz, 266 g; GI= 66 (Medium); GL= 6.6 (Low); Net carb= 10 g

Apple Cider ☛ Serving size= 12 fl oz, 355 g; GI= 40 (Low); GL= 8.4 (Low); Net carb= 21 g

Barbera ☛ Serving size= 1 fl oz, 29.4 g; GI= 7 (Low); GL= 0.1 (Low); Net carb= 0.8 g

Bottled Water ☛ Serving size= 8 fl oz, 266 g; GI= 0 (Low); GL= 0 (Low); Net carb= 0 g

Cola Or Pepper-Type, Low Calorie With Aspartame Contains Caffeine ☛ Serving size= 8 fl oz, 266 g; GI= 54 (Low); GL= 0.4 (Low); Net carb= 0.8 g

Limeade High Caffeine ☛ Serving size= 8 fl oz, 266 g; GI= 68 (Medium); GL= 7.4 (Low); Net carb= 10.9 g

Carbonated Drink, Other Than Cola Or Pepper, Low Calorie With Aspartame ☛ Serving size= 8 fl oz, 266 g; GI= 54 (Low); GL= 0 (Low); Net carb= 0 g

Chicory Beverage ☛ Serving size= 8 fl oz, 266 g; GI= 9 (Low); GL= 0.3 (Low); Net carb= 3.8 g

Chocolate Almond Milk ☛ Serving size= 4 fl oz, 133 g; GI= 35 (Low); GL= 4.2 (Low); Net carb= 11.9 g

Citrus Green Tea ☛ Serving size= 8 fl oz, 266 g; GI= 0 (Low); GL= 0 (Low); Net carb= 0.8 g

Coconut Water—Ready-To-Drink—Unsweetened ☛ Serving size= 8 fl oz, 266 g; GI= 41 (Low); GL= 4.6 (Low); Net carb= 11.3 g

Coffee ☛ Serving size= 1 fl oz, 29.6 g; GI= 0 (Low); GL= 0 (Low); Net carb= 0 g

Coffee Instant, Chicory ☛ Serving size= 1 fl oz, 29.9 g; GI= 7 (Low); GL= 0 (Low); Net carb= 0.2 g

Coffee Instant, Chicory, Powder ☛ Serving size= 1 tsp, rounded, 1.8 g; GI= 89 (High); GL= 1.2 (Low); Net carb= 1.4 g

Coffee Instant, Decaffeinated Powder ☛ Serving size= 1 tsp rounded, 1.8 g; GI= 89 (High); GL= 1.2 (Low); Net carb= 1.4 g

Coffee Instant, Mocha Sweetened ☛ Serving size= 1 serving 2 tbsp, 13 g; GI= 89 (High); GL= 8.4 (Low); Net carb= 9.4 g

Coffee Instant, Reconstituted ☛ Serving size= 1 fl oz, 30 g; GI= 0 (Low); GL= 0 (Low); Net carb= 0.2 g

Coffee Instant, Regular Half The Caffeine ☛ Serving size= 1 tsp, 1 g; GI= 89 (High); GL= 0.6 (Low); Net carb= 0.7 g

Coffee Instant, Regular Powder ☛ Serving size= 1 tsp, 1 g; GI= 89 (High); GL= 0.7 (Low); Net carb= 0.8 g

Coffee, Bottled or canned, Light ☛ Serving size= 1 fl oz, 30 g; GI= 21 (Low); GL= 0.4 (Low); Net carb= 1.8 g

Coffee, Brewed—Espresso Restaurant-Made Decaffeinated ☛ Serving size= 1 fl oz, 29.6 g; GI= 0 (Low); GL= 0 (Low); Net carb= 0.5 g

Coffee, Cafe Con Leche ☛ Serving size= 1 fl oz, 31 g; GI= 5 (Low); GL= 0.1 (Low); Net carb= 1.7 g

Coffee, Cafe Con Leche Decaffeinated ☛ Serving size= 1 fl oz, 31 g; GI= 21 (Low); GL= 0.4 (Low); Net carb= 1.8 g

Coffee, Cafe Mocha ☛ Serving size= 1 fl oz, 31 g; GI= 21 (Low); GL= 0.7 (Low); Net carb= 3.1 g

Coffee, Cappuccino ☛ Serving size= 1 fl oz, 30 g; GI= 33 (Low); GL= 0.3 (Low); Net carb= 0.8 g

Coffee, Cuban ☛ Serving size= 1 fl oz, 31 g; GI= 41 (Low); GL= 1 (Low); Net carb= 2.4 g

Coffee, Espresso ☛ Serving size= 1 fl oz, 29.6 g; GI= 0 (Low); GL= 0 (Low); Net carb= 0.5 g

Coffee, Latte ☛ Serving size= 1 fl oz, 30 g; GI= 21 (Low); GL= 0.3 (Low); Net carb= 1.3 g

Coffee, Macchiato ☛ Serving size= 1 fl oz, 30 g; GI= 21 (Low); GL= 0.2 (Low); Net carb= 0.8 g

Coffee, Turkish ☛ Serving size= 1 fl oz, 31 g; GI= 51 (Low); GL= 1 (Low); Net carb= 2 g

Diet Cola ☛ Serving size= 8 fl oz, 266 g; GI= 41 (Low); GL= 5.6 (Low); Net carb= 13.7 g

Diet Pepper Cola ☛ Serving size= 8 fl oz, 266 g; GI= 11 (Low); GL= 0 (Low); Net carb= 0.3 g

Energy Drink Amp Sugar Free ☛ Serving size= 8 fl oz, 266 g; GI= 0 (Low); GL= 0 (Low); Net carb= 2.7 g

Energy Drink, Low Carb Monster ☛ Serving size= 8 fl oz, 266 g; GI= 15 (Low); GL= 0.6 (Low); Net carb= 3.7 g

Energy Drink, Red Bull Sugar Free ☛ Serving size= 8 fl oz, 266 g; GI= 0 (Low); GL= 0 (Low); Net carb= 1.9 g

Energy Drink, Rockstar Sugar Free ☛ Serving size= 8 fl oz, 266 g; GI= 0 (Low); GL= 0 (Low); Net carb= 1.9 g

Energy Drink, Sugar Free ☛ Serving size= 8 fl oz, 266 g; GI= 0 (Low); GL= 0 (Low); Net carb= 1.1 g

Energy Drink, Vault Zero Sugar-Free Citrus Flavor ☛ Serving size= 8 fl oz, 266 g; GI= 0 (Low); GL= 0 (Low); Net carb= 1.9 g

Fruit Flavored Smoothie Drink Frozen Light No Dairy ☛ Serving size= 8 fl oz, 266 g; GI= 68 (Medium); GL= 5.8 (Low); Net carb= 8.5 g

Fruit Juice Drink—Diet ☛ Serving size= 8 fl oz, 266 g; GI= 0 (Low); GL= 0 (Low); Net carb= 1.3 g

Green Tea ☛ Serving size= 16 fl oz, 473 g; GI= 0 (Low); GL= 0 (Low); Net carb= 0 g

Lemonade—Powder Made With Water ☛ Serving size= 8 fl oz, 266 g; GI= 68 (Medium); GL= 6.5 (Low); Net carb= 9.5 g

Mixed Berry Powerade Zero ☛ Serving size= 12 fl oz, 360 g; GI= 0 (Low); GL= 0 (Low); Net carb= 0.5 g

Rich Chocolate Powder ☛ Serving size= 2 tbsp, 11 g; GI= 89 (High); GL= 9.1 (Low); Net carb= 10.2 g

Soy Protein Powder ☛ Serving size= 1 scoop, 44 g; GI= 47 (Low); GL= 9.1 (Low); Net carb= 19.3 g

Sweetened Vanilla Almond Milk ☛ Serving size= 8 fl oz, 266 g; GI= 33 (Low); GL= 5.4 (Low); Net carb= 16.5 g

Tap Water ☛ Serving size= 8 fl oz, 266 g; GI= 0 (Low); GL= 0 (Low); Net carb= 0 g

Tea Green, Brewed ☛ Serving size= 1 cup, 245 g; GI= 0 (Low); GL= 0 (Low); Net carb= 0 g

Tea Black , Brewed) ☛ Serving size= 1 fl oz, 29.6 g; GI= 0 (Low); GL= 0 (Low); Net carb= 0.1 g

Tea Black, Ready To Drink ☛ Serving size= 16 fl oz, 473 g; GI= 0 (Low); GL= 0 (Low); Net carb= 0 g

Tea Black, Ready-To-Drink—Lemon Diet ☛ Serving size= 1 cup, 265 g; GI= 0 (Low); GL= 0 (Low); Net carb= 0.6 g

Tea Black, Ready-To-Drink—Peach Diet ☛ Serving size= 1 cup, 268 g; GI= 0 (Low); GL= 0 (Low); Net carb= 0.7 g

Tea Herb, Other Than Chamomile Brewed ☛ Serving size= 1 fl oz, 29.6 g; GI= 0 (Low); GL= 0 (Low); Net carb= 0.1 g

Tea Herb, Brewed—Chamomile ☛ Serving size= 1 fl oz, 29.6 g; GI= 0 (Low); GL= 0 (Low); Net carb= 0.1 g

Tea Herb, Hibiscus Brewed ☛ Serving size= 8 fl oz, 237 g; GI= 0 (Low); GL= 0 (Low); Net carb= 0 g

Whey Protein Powder ☛ Serving size= 2 scoop, 39 g; GI= 47 (Low); GL= 3.3 (Low); Net carb= 7 g

# CONDIMENTS, OILS & SAUCES

Alfredo Sauce ☞ Serving size= ¼ cup, 62 g; GI= 27 (Low); GL= 0.4 (Low); Net carb= 1.6 g

Beef Tallow ☞ Serving size= 1 tbsp, 15 g; GI= 0 (Low); GL= 0 (Low); Net carb= 0 g

Clarified Butter ☞ Serving size= 1 tbsp, 15 g; GI= 0 (Low); GL= 0 (Low); Net carb= 0 g

Cocktail sauce ☞ Serving size= ¼ cup, 62 g; GI= 38 (Low); GL= 6.8 (Low); Net carb= 18 g

Dressing—Blue or roquefort ☞ Serving size= 2 tbsp, 30 g; GI= 50 (Low); GL= 4.1 (Low); Net carb= 8.1 g

Dressing—Blue or roquefort, low-calorie ☞ Serving size= 2 tbsp, 30 g; GI= 5 (Low); GL= 0 (Low); Net carb= 0.9 g

Dressing—Blue or roquefort, reduced calorie ☞ Serving size= 2 tbsp, 30 g; GI= 5 (Low); GL= 0 (Low); Net carb= 0.9 g

Dressing—Blue or roquefort, reduced calorie, fat-free ☞ Serving size= 2 tbsp, 30 g; GI= 5 (Low); GL= 0 (Low); Net carb= 0.9 g

Dressing—Caesar ☞ Serving size= ¼ cup, 62 g; GI= 50 (Low); GL= 0.8 (Low); Net carb= 1.6 g

Dressing—Caesar, low-calorie ☞ Serving size= ¼ cup, 62 g; GI= 5 (Low); GL= 0 (Low); Net carb= 0.2 g

Dressing—Coleslaw ☞ Serving size= ¼ cup, 62 g; GI= 50 (Low); GL= 1.2 (Low); Net carb= 2.3 g

Dressing—Coleslaw, reduced calorie ☞ Serving size= ¼ cup, 62 g; GI= 5 (Low); GL= 0 (Low); Net carb= 0 g

Dressing—Cream cheese ☞ Serving size= 2 tbsp, 30 g; GI= 50 (Low); GL= 0.5 (Low); Net carb= 1 g

Dressing—Feta Cheese ☞ Serving size= ¼ cup, 62 g; GI= 50 (Low); GL= 0.7 (Low); Net carb= 1.4 g

Dressing—French ☞ Serving size= 2 tbsp, 30 g; GI= 50 (Low); GL= 4.5 (Low); Net carb= 9 g

Dressing—French, reduced calorie ☞ Serving size= 2 tbsp, 30 g; GI= 50 (Low); GL= 1.9 (Low); Net carb= 3.8 g

Dressing—French, reduced calorie, fat free ☞ Serving size= 2 tbsp, 30 g; GI= 50 (Low); GL= 1.9 (Low); Net carb= 3.8 g

Dressing—Green Goddess ☞ Serving size= 2 tbsp, 30 g; GI= 50 (Low); GL= 1.2 (Low); Net carb= 2.4 g

Dressing—Honey mustard ☞ Serving size= 2 tbsp, 30 g; GI= 50 (Low); GL= 4.2 (Low); Net carb= 8.4 g

Dressing—Honey mustard ☞ Serving size= ¼ cup, 62 g; GI= (Low); GL= 0 (Low); Net carb= 16.8 g

Dressing—Italian dressing ☞ Serving size= 2 tbsp, 30 g; GI= 50 (Low); GL= 1.1 (Low); Net carb= 2.2 g

Dressing—Italian, diet or reduced calorie ☞ Serving size= 2 tbsp, 30 g; GI= 5 (Low); GL= 0 (Low); Net carb= 0.4 g

Dressing—Italian, diet or reduced calorie, fat free ☞ Serving size= 2 tbsp, 30 g; GI= 5 (Low); GL= 0 (Low); Net carb= 0.4 g

Dressing—Italian, reduced calorie ☞ Serving size= 2 tbsp, 30 g; GI= 5 (Low); GL= 0 (Low); Net carb= 0.4 g

Dressing—Korean ☞ Serving size= ¼ cup, 62 g; GI= 50 (Low); GL= 1.9 (Low); Net carb= 3.7 g

Dressing—Mayonnaise-type salad, cholesterol-free ☞ Serving size= 2 tbsp, 30 g; GI= 50 (Low); GL= 3 (Low); Net carb= 6 g

Dressing—Mayonnaise-type salad, diet ☞ Serving size= 2 tbsp, 30 g; GI= 50 (Low); GL= 1.1 (Low); Net carb= 2.2 g

Dressing—Milk, vinegar based ☞ Serving size= 2 tbsp, 30 g; GI= 50 (Low); GL= 1 (Low); Net carb= 1.9 g

Dressing—Peppercorn ☞ Serving size= 2 tbsp, 30 g; GI= 50 (Low); GL= 1 (Low); Net carb= 2 g

Dressing—Peppercorn ☞ Serving size= ¼ cup, 62 g; GI= 50 (Low); GL= 2 (Low); Net carb= 4 g

Dressing—Poppy seed ☞ Serving size= ¼ cup, 62 g; GI= 50 (Low); GL= 6.2 (Low); Net carb= 12.4 g

Dressing—Poppy seed ☞ Serving size= 2 tbsp, 30 g; GI= 50 (Low); GL= 3.1 (Low); Net carb= 6.2 g

Dressing—Rice ☞ Serving size= ¼ cup, 62 g; GI= 64 (Low); GL= 6.7 (Low); Net carb= 10.5 g

Dressing—Rice ☞ Serving size= 2 tbsp, 30 g; GI= 64 (Low); GL= 3.4 (Low); Net carb= 5.3 g

Dressing—Russian ☞ Serving size= ¼ cup, 62 g; GI= 50 (Low); GL= 9.7 (Low); Net carb= 19.3 g

Dressing—Russian ☞ Serving size= 2 tbsp, 30 g; GI= 50 (Low); GL= 4.8 (Low); Net carb= 9.6 g

Dressing—Salad, common ☛ Serving size= ¼ cup, 62 g; GI= 50 (Low); GL= 2.8 (Low); Net carb= 5.6 g

Dressing—Salad, common ☛ Serving size= 2 tbsp, 30 g; GI= 50 (Low); GL= 1.4 (Low); Net carb= 2.8 g

Dressing—Sesame ☛ Serving size= ¼ cup, 62 g; GI= 50 (Low); GL= 7.4 (Low); Net carb= 14.8 g

Dressing—Sesame ☛ Serving size= 2 tbsp, 30 g; GI= 50 (Low); GL= 3.7 (Low); Net carb= 7.4 g

Dressing—Sweet and sour ☛ Serving size= ¼ cup, 62 g; GI= 50 (Low); GL= 1.2 (Low); Net carb= 2.4 g

Dressing—Thousand Island Regular ☛ Serving size= 2 tbsp, 30 g; GI= 50 (Low); GL= 1.5 (Low); Net carb= 2.9 g

Dressing—Thousand Island Regular ☛ Serving size= ¼ cup, 62 g; GI= 50 (Low); GL= 2.9 (Low); Net carb= 5.8 g

Dressing—Vinegar based ☛ Serving size= ¼ cup, 62 g; GI= 50 (Low); GL= 0.8 (Low); Net carb= 1.6 g

Dressing—Yogurt ☛ Serving size= ¼ cup, 62 g; GI= 50 (Low); GL= 1.9 (Low); Net carb= 3.8 g

Dressing—Yogurt ☛ Serving size= 2 tbsp, 30 g; GI= 50 (Low); GL= 1 (Low); Net carb= 1.9 g

Duck Fat ☛ Serving size= 2 tbsp, 30 g; GI= 0 (Low); GL= 0 (Low); Net carb= 0 g

Mayonnaise (mean value) ☛ Serving size= 2 tbsp, 30 g; GI= 50 (Low); GL= 1.2 (Low); Net carb= 2.4 g

Mayonnaise—made with tofu ☛ Serving size= 2 tbsp, 30 g; GI= 50 (Low); GL= 0.3 (Low); Net carb= 0.6 g

Mustard greens (mean value) ☛ Serving size= 2 tbsp, 30 g; GI= 32 (Low); GL= 0.2 (Low); Net carb= 0.5 g

Mustard pickles ☞ Serving size= 2 tbsp, 30 g; GI= 32 (Low); GL= 2.4 (Low); Net carb= 7.5 g

Oil—Avocado ☞ Serving size= 2 tbsp, 30 g; GI= 0 (Low); GL= 0 (Low); Net carb= 0 g

Oil—Canola ☞ Serving size= 2 tbsp, 30 g; GI= 0 (Low); GL= 0 (Low); Net carb= 0 g

Oil—Coconut ☞ Serving size= 2 tbsp, 30 g; GI= 0 (Low); GL= 0 (Low); Net carb= 0 g

Oil—Corn ☞ Serving size= 2 tbsp, 30 g; GI= 0 (Low); GL= 0 (Low); Net carb= 0 g

Oil—Extra-virgin olive ☞ Serving size= 2 tbsp, 30 g; GI= 0 (Low); GL= 0 (Low); Net carb= 0 g

Oil—Flaxseed ☞ Serving size= 2 tbsp, 30 g; GI= 0 (Low); GL= 0 (Low); Net carb= 0 g

Oil—Grapeseed ☞ Serving size= 2 tbsp, 30 g; GI= 0 (Low); GL= 0 (Low); Net carb= 0 g

Oil—Hazelnut ☞ Serving size= 2 tbsp, 30 g; GI= 0 (Low); GL= 0 (Low); Net carb= 0 g

Oil—Hemp seed ☞ Serving size= 2 tbsp, 30 g; GI= 0 (Low); GL= 0 (Low); Net carb= 0 g

Oil—Macadamia Nut ☞ Serving size= 2 tbsp, 30 g; GI= 0 (Low); GL= 0 (Low); Net carb= 0 g

Oil—Olive ☞ Serving size= 2 tbsp, 30 g; GI= 0 (Low); GL= 0 (Low); Net carb= 0 g

Oil—Palm ☞ Serving size= 2 tbsp, 30 g; GI= 0 (Low); GL= 0 (Low); Net carb= 0 g

Oil—Peanut ☞ Serving size= 2 tbsp, 30 g; GI= 0 (Low); GL= 0 (Low); Net carb= 0 g

Oil—Rice Bran ☞ Serving size= 2 tbsp, 30 g; GI= 0 (Low); GL= 0 (Low); Net carb= 0 g

Oil—Sesame ☞ Serving size= 2 tbsp, 30 g; GI= 0 (Low); GL= 0 (Low); Net carb= 0 g

Oil—Sunflower ☞ Serving size= 2 tbsp, 30 g; GI= 0 (Low); GL= 0 (Low); Net carb= 0 g

Oil—Vegetable ☞ Serving size= 2 tbsp, 30 g; GI= 0 (Low); GL= 0 (Low); Net carb= 0 g

Oil—Walnut ☞ Serving size= 2 tbsp, 30 g; GI= 0 (Low); GL= 0 (Low); Net carb= 0 g

Vinegar, sugar, and water dressing ☞ Serving size= 2 tbsp, 30 g; GI= 0 (Low); GL= 0 (Low); Net carb= 0 g

# DAIRY AND SOY ALTERNATIVES

Butter-vegetable oil blend ☞ Serving size: 1 tsp (4.7 g); GI= 50 (Low); GL= 0.3 (Low); Net carb= 0.6 g

Butter, minimally processed ☞ Serving size: 1 tsp (4.7 g); GI= 50 (Low); GL= 0.3 (Low); Net carb= 0.6 g

Butter, stick, unsalted ☞ Serving size: 1 tsp (4.7 g); GI= 50 (Low); GL= 0.3 (Low); Net carb= 0.6 g

Butter, whipped, stick, unsalted ☞ Serving size: 1 tsp (4.7 g); GI= 50 (Low); GL= 0.3 (Low); Net carb= 0.6 g

Butter, whipped, tub, unsalted ☞ Serving size: 1 tsp (4.7 g); GI= 50 (Low); GL= 0.3 (Low); Net carb= 0.6 g

Buttermilk, fluid ☞ Serving size: 1 cup (245 g); GI= 29.5 (Low); GL= 3.6 (Low); Net carb= 12.2 g

Carry-out milk shake, chocolate ☞ Serving size: 1 cup (245 g); GI= 44 (Low); GL= 5.4 (Low); Net carb= 12.3 g

Carry-out milk shake, flavors other than chocolate ☞ Serving size: 1 cup (245 g); GI= 44 (Low); GL= 5.4 (Low); Net carb= 12.3 g

Cheese—Amercican style ☛ Serving size: 1 oz (28.35 g); GI= 27 (Low); GL= 0.2 (Low); Net carb= 0.7 g

Cheese—Blue ☛ Serving size: 1 oz (28.35 g); GI= 0.0 (Low); GL= 0 (Low); Net carb= 0 g

Cheese—camembert ☛ Serving size: 1 oz (28.35 g); GI= 25 (Low); GL= 0.2 (Low); Net carb= 0.8 g

Cheese—cheddar ☛ Serving size: 1 oz (28.35 g); GI= 27 (Low); GL= 0.2 (Low); Net carb= 0.7 g

Cheese—Colby ☛ Serving size: 1 oz (28.35 g); GI= 27 (Low); GL= 0.2 (Low); Net carb= 0.7 g

Cheese—cottage, minimally processed ☛ Serving size: 1 oz (28.35 g); GI= 29.5 (Low); GL= 0.3 (Low); Net carb= 1 g

Cheese—cottage, with fruit ☛ Serving size: 1 oz (28.35 g); GI= 42.5 (Low); GL= 0.4 (Low); Net carb= 0.9 g

Cheese—cream ☛ Serving size: 1 oz (28.35 g); GI= 27 (Low); GL= 2.3 (Low); Net carb= 8.5 g

Cheese—Edam ☛ Serving size: 1 oz (28.35 g); GI= 27 (Low); GL= 0.2 (Low); Net carb= 0.7 g

Cheese—Feta ☛ Serving size: 1 oz (28.35 g); GI= 27 (Low); GL= 0.2 (Low); Net carb= 0.7 g

Cheese—Fontina ☛ Serving size: 1 oz (28.35 g); GI= 27 (Low); GL= 0.2 (Low); Net carb= 0.7 g

Cheese—goat ☛ Serving size: 1 oz (28.35 g); GI= 27 (Low); GL= 0.2 (Low); Net carb= 0.7 g

Cheese—Gouda ☛ Serving size: 1 oz (28.35 g); GI= 27 (Low); GL= 0.2 (Low); Net carb= 0.7 g

Cheese—Gruyere ☛ Serving size: 1 oz (28.35 g); GI= 27 (Low); GL= 0.2 (Low); Net carb= 0.7 g

Cheese—halloumi ☞ Serving size: 1 oz (28.35 g); GI= 0.0 (Low); GL= 0 (Low); Net carb= 0 g

Cheese—havarti ☞ Serving size: 1 oz (28.35 g); GI= 0.0 (Low); GL= 0 (Low); Net carb= 0 g

Cheese—Limburger ☞ Serving size: 1 oz (28.35 g); GI= 27 (Low); GL= 0.2 (Low); Net carb= 0.7 g

Cheese—Manchego ☞ Serving size: 1 oz (28.35 g); GI= 27 (Low); GL= 0.2 (Low); Net carb= 0.7 g

Cheese—Monterey ☞ Serving size: 1 oz (28.35 g); GI= 27 (Low); GL= 0.2 (Low); Net carb= 0.7 g

Cheese—mozzarella ☞ Serving size: 1 oz (28.35 g); GI= 27 (Low); GL= 0.2 (Low); Net carb= 0.7 g

Cheese—Muenster ☞ Serving size: 1 oz (28.35 g); GI= 27 (Low); GL= 0.2 (Low); Net carb= 0.7 g

Cheese—Parmesan ☞ Serving size: 1 oz (28.35 g); GI= 27 (Low); GL= 0.2 (Low); Net carb= 0.7 g

Cheese—Pecorino Romano ☞ Serving size: 1 oz (28.35 g); GI= 0.0 (Low); GL= 0 (Low); Net carb= 0 g

Cheese—Provolone ☞ Serving size: 1 oz (28.35 g); GI= 27 (Low); GL= 0.2 (Low); Net carb= 0.7 g

Cheese—Ricotta ☞ Serving size: 1 oz (28.35 g); GI= 27 (Low); GL= 0.2 (Low); Net carb= 0.7 g

Cheese—Roquefort ☞ Serving size: 1 oz (28.35 g); GI= 0.0 (Low); GL= 0 (Low); Net carb= 0 g

Cheese—Swiss ☞ Serving size: 1 oz (28.35 g); GI= 27 (Low); GL= 0.2 (Low); Net carb= 0.7 g

Cow's Milk, whole, skim or reduced fat ☞ Serving size: 1 cup (245 g); GI= 40 (Low); GL= 4.8 (Low); Net carb= 12 g

Cream cheese ☛ Serving size: 1 oz (28.35 g); GI= 0.0 (Low); GL= 0 (Low); Net carb= 0 g

Cream—light, fluid ☛ Serving size: 1 oz (28.35 g); GI= 27 (Low); GL= 2.3 (Low); Net carb= 8.5 g

Cream—light, whipped, and unsweetened ☛ Serving size: 1 oz (28.35 g); GI= 27 (Low); GL= 2.3 (Low); Net carb= 8.5 g

Custard homemade ☛ Serving size: ½ cup (116 g); GI= 29 (Low); GL= 6.7 (Low); Net carb= 23.1 g

Custard—Puerto Rican style ☛ Serving size: ½ cup (116 g); GI= 38 (Low); GL= 8.8 (Low); Net carb= 23.2 g

Dip, cheese—chili con queso ☛ Serving size: 1 oz (28.35 g); GI= 27 (Low); GL= 9.4 (Low); Net carb= 34.8 g

Ghee ☛ Serving size: 1 tsp (4.7 g); GI= 0.0 (Low); GL= 0 (Low); Net carb= 0 g

Cheese—Goat ☛ Serving size: 1 oz (28.35 g); GI= 27 (Low); GL= 0.2 (Low); Net carb= 0.7 g

Goat's Milk whole ☛ Serving size: 1 cup (245 g); GI= 40 (Low); GL= 4.4 (Low); Net carb= 11 g

Goat's milk yoghurt ☛ Serving size: 8 oz (225 g); GI= 25 (Low); GL= 2.75 (Low); Net carb= 11 g

Ice cream—average value ☛ Serving size: 1 scoop ( 72 g)

; GI= 64.5 (Medium); GL= 7.9 (Low); Net carb= 12.2 g

Imitation cheese, American type ☛ Serving size: 1 oz (28.35 g); GI= 27 (Low); GL= 1.8 (Low); Net carb= 6.7 g

Imitation cheese, cheddar ☛ Serving size: 1 oz (28.35 g); GI= 27 (Low); GL= 1.8 (Low); Net carb= 6.7 g

Imitation cheese, Edam ☛ Serving size: 1 oz (28.35 g); GI= 27 (Low); GL= 1.8 (Low); Net carb= 6.7 g

Imitation cheese, Mozzarella ☛ Serving size: 1 oz (28.35 g); GI= 27 (Low); GL= 1.8 (Low); Net carb= 6.7 g

Kefir ☛ Serving size: 1 cup (245 g); GI= 32 (Low); GL= 0.7 (Low); Net carb= 2.2 g

Margarine-based spread, unsalted ☛ Serving size: 1 tsp (4.7 g); GI= 50 (Low); GL= 0 (Low); Net carb= 0 g

Margarine—stick, unsalted ☛ Serving size: 1 tsp (4.7 g); GI= 50 (Low); GL= 0 (Low); Net carb= 0 g

Margarine—tub, unsalted ☛ Serving size: 1 tsp (4.7 g); GI= 50 (Low); GL= 0 (Low); Net carb= 0 g

Margarine—whipped, tub, unsalted ☛ Serving size: 1 tsp (4.7 g); GI= 50 (Low); GL= 0 (Low); Net carb= 0 g

Milk beverage—nonfat dry milk , flavors other than chocolate and low-calorie sweetener ☛ Serving size: 1 cup (245 g); GI= 24 (Low); GL= 2.6 (Low); Net carb= 10.8 g

Milk beverage—nonfat dry milk, chocolate and low calorie sweetener ☛ Serving size: 1 cup (245 g); GI= 24 (Low); GL= 2.6 (Low); Net carb= 10.8 g

Milk beverage—whole milk, flavors other than chocolate ☛ Serving size: 1 cup (245 g); GI= 35 (Low); GL= 3.9 (Low); Net carb= 11.1 g

Milk dessert—frozen, chocolate (no butterfat) ☛ Serving size: ½ cup (68 g); GI= 61 (Medium); GL= 6.6 (Low); Net carb= 10.8 g

Milk dessert—frozen, flavors other than chocolate ☛ Serving size: ½ cup (68 g); GI= 61 (Medium); GL= 6.6 (Low); Net carb= 10.8 g

Milk dessert—frozen, low-calorie sweetener ☛ Serving size: ½ cup (68 g); GI= 50 (Low); GL= 5.4 (Low); Net carb= 10.8 g

Milk dessert—frozen, lowfat, flavors other than chocolate ☛ Serving size: ½ cup (68 g); GI= 50 (Low); GL= 5.4 (Low); Net carb= 10.8 g

Milk lactose—free ☛ Serving size: 1 cup (245 g); GI= 40 (Low); GL= 6 (Low); Net carb= 15 g

Milk made from soy protein ☛ Serving size: 1 cup (245 g); GI= 50 (Low); GL= 7.4 (Low); Net carb= 14.8 g

Milk—chocolate, average value ☛ Serving size: 1 cup (245 g); GI= 37 (Low); GL= 9.1 (Low); Net carb= 24.6 g

Milk—chocolate, whole ☛ Serving size: 1 cup (245 g); GI= 36 (Low); GL= 8.8 (Low); Net carb= 24.4 g

Milk—dry, reconstituted, average value ☛ Serving size: 1 cup (245 g); GI= 32 (Low); GL= 3.8 (Low); Net carb= 11.9 g

Milk—goat's, fluid, whole ☛ Serving size: 1 cup (245 g); GI= 27 (Low); GL= 3.24 (Low); Net carb= 12 g

Milk—imitation, fluid, soy based ☛ Serving size: 1 cup (245 g); GI= 40 (Low); GL= 4.8 (Low); Net carb= 12 g

Milk—malted, fortified, chocolate, made with milk ☛ Serving size: 1 cup (245 g); GI= 45 (Low); GL= 5.4 (Low); Net carb= 12 g

Milk—soy, dry, reconstituted, not baby's ☛ Serving size: 1 cup (245 g); GI= 40 (Low); GL= 5.9 (Low); Net carb= 14.8 g

Milk—soy, ready-to-drink, not baby's ☛ Serving size: 1 cup (245 g); GI= 40 (Low); GL= 5.9 (Low); Net carb= 14.8 g

Milk, almond ☛ Serving size: 1 cup (245 g); GI= 25 (Low); GL= 2 (Low); Net carb= 8 g

Milk, coconut ☛ Serving size: 1 cup (245 g); GI= 41 (Low); GL= 6 (Low); Net carb= 14.6 g

Milk, hemp ☛ Serving size: 1 cup (245 g); GI= 0.0 (Low); GL= 0 (Low); Net carb= 0 g

Milk, soy, beans ☛ Serving size: 1 cup (245 g); GI= 41 (Low); GL= 6 (Low); Net carb= 14.6 g

Pudding—pumpkin ☞ Serving size: 4 oz (120 g); GI= 47 (Low); GL= 9.4 (Low); Net carb= 20 g

Queso—Anejo (aged cheese) ☞ Serving size: 1 oz (28.35 g); GI= 27 (Low); GL= 0.2 (Low); Net carb= 0.7 g

Queso—Asadero ☞ Serving size: 1 oz (28.35 g); GI= 27 (Low); GL= 0.2 (Low); Net carb= 0.7 g

Queso—Chihuahua ☞ Serving size: 1 oz (28.35 g); GI= 27 (Low); GL= 0.2 (Low); Net carb= 0.7 g

Queso—Fresco ☞ Serving size: 1 oz (28.35 g); GI= 27 (Low); GL= 0.5 (Low); Net carb= 1.9 g

Soy Cheese ☞ Serving size: 1 oz (28.35 g); GI= 40 (Low); GL= 2.7 (Low); Net carb= 6.8 g

Traditional Greek yoghurt ☞ Serving size: 1 cup (245 g); GI= 0.0 (Low); GL= 0 (Low); Net carb= 0 g

Yoghurt—lactose free ☞ Serving size: 1 cup (245 g); GI= 50 (Low); GL= 4.9 (Low); Net carb= 9.8 g

Yoghurt—natural low-fat ☞ Serving size: 1 cup (245 g); GI= 50 (Low); GL= 4.9 (Low); Net carb= 9.8 g

Yoghurt—natural regular-fat ☞ Serving size: 1 cup (245 g); GI= 50 (Low); GL= 4.9 (Low); Net carb= 9.8 g

Yogurt—chocolate, nonfat milk ☞ Serving size: 1 cup (245 g); GI= 32 (Low); GL= 3.1 (Low); Net carb= 9.7 g

Yogurt—frozen, chocolate ☞ Serving size: 1 cup (245 g); GI= 50 (Low); GL= 4.9 (Low); Net carb= 9.8 g

Yogurt—frozen, flavors other than chocolate ☞ Serving size: 1 cup (245 g); GI= 50 (Low); GL= 4.9 (Low); Net carb= 9.8 g

Yogurt—fruit variety ☞ Serving size: 1 cup (245 g); GI= 31 (Low); GL= 3 (Low); Net carb= 9.7 g

Yogurt—plain ☛ Serving size: 1 cup (245 g); GI= 36 (Low); GL= 3.5 (Low); Net carb= 9.7 g

Yogurt—vanilla, lemon, or coffee flavor, whole milk ☛ Serving size: 1 cup (245 g); GI= 27 (Low); GL= 2.6 (Low); Net carb= 9.6 g

# LEGUMS AND BEANS

Adzuki Beans 🖝 Serving size= ½ cup, 150 g; GI= 33 (Low); GL= 8.6 (Low); Net carb= 26.2 g

Adzuki Beans—Mature Seed Cooked 🖝 Serving size= ½ cup, 150 g; GI= 33 (Low); GL= 8.6 (Low); Net carb= 26.2 g

Baked Beans 🖝 Serving size= ½ cup, 150 g; GI= 40 (Low); GL= 9.7 (Low); Net carb= 24.2 g

Baked Beans—Canned No Added Sugar 🖝 Serving size= ½ cup, 150 g; GI= 40 (Low); GL= 9 (Low); Net carb= 22.5 g

Bayo Beans—Canned Drained and cooked 🖝 Serving size= ½ cup, 150 g; GI= 30 (Low); GL= 6.4 (Low); Net carb= 21.4 g

Bayo Beans—Dry Cooked 🖝 Serving size= ½ cup, 150 g; GI= 30 (Low); GL= 6.7 (Low); Net carb= 22.3 g

Black Beans—Mature Seeds Cooked 🖝 Serving size= ½ cup, 150 g; GI= 30 (Low); GL= 6.8 (Low); Net carb= 22.5 g

Black Beans—Turtle Mature Seeds Canned 🖝 Serving size= ½ cup, 150 g; GI= 41 (Low); GL= 5.9 (Low); Net carb= 14.5 g

Black Beans—Turtle Mature Seeds Cooked ☞ Serving size= ½ cup, 150 g; GI= 41 (Low); GL= 9.9 (Low); Net carb= 24.1 g

Broad Beans (Fava) ☞ Serving size= ½ cup, 150 g; GI= 40 (Low); GL= 8.6 (Low); Net carb= 21.4 g

Broad beans (Fava)—Mature Seeds Canned ☞ Serving size= ½ cup, 150 g; GI= 40 (Low); GL= 5.2 (Low); Net carb= 13.1 g

Broad beans (Fava)—Mature Seeds Cooked ☞ Serving size= ½ cup, 150 g; GI= 40 (Low); GL= 8.6 (Low); Net carb= 21.4 g

California Red Kidney Beans ☞ Serving size= ½ cup, 150 g; GI= 33 (Low); GL= 6.5 (Low); Net carb= 19.7 g

Chickpeas (Garbanzo)—Canned Drained, Cooked ☞ Serving size= ½ cup, 150 g; GI= 36 (Low); GL= 8.2 (Low); Net carb= 22.7 g

Chickpeas (Garbanzo)—Dry Cooked ☞ Serving size= ½ cup, 150 g; GI= 36 (Low); GL= 9.9 (Low); Net carb= 27.4 g

Chickpeas (Garbanzo)—Mature Seeds Canned Drained Rinsed ☞ Serving size= ½ cup, 150 g; GI= 36 (Low); GL= 8.9 (Low); Net carb= 24.9 g

Chickpeas (Garbanzo)—Stewed With Pig's Feet Puerto Rican Style ☞ Serving size= ½ cup, 150 g; GI= 36 (Low); GL= 3.6 (Low); Net carb= 9.9 g

Cowpeas—Dry Cooked ☞ Serving size= ½ cup, 150 g; GI= 50 (Low); GL= 9.8 (Low); Net carb= 19.7 g

Cowpeas—Mature Seeds Canned Plain ☞ Serving size= ½ cup, 150 g; GI= 50 (Low); GL= 7.7 (Low); Net carb= 15.5 g

Cowpeas—Mature Seeds Canned With Pork ☞ Serving size= ½ cup, 150 g; GI= 50 (Low); GL= 9.9 (Low); Net carb= 19.8 g

Edamame ☞ Serving size= ½ cup, 150 g; GI= 20 (Low); GL= 1.1 (Low); Net carb= 5.6 g

Extra Firm Tofu ☞ Serving size= ½ cup, 150 g; GI= 15 (Low); GL= 0.2 (Low); Net carb= 1.2 g

French Beans—Mature Seeds Cooked ☞ Serving size= ½ cup, 150 g; GI= 21 (Low); GL= 4.6 (Low); Net carb= 21.9 g

Green Or Yellow Split Peas—Dry Cooked ☞ Serving size= ½ cup, 150 g; GI= 33 (Low); GL= 6.3 (Low); Net carb= 19 g

Green Soybeans ☞ Serving size= ½ cup, 150 g; GI= 18 (Low); GL= 1.8 (Low); Net carb= 10.3 g

Hummus (Commercial) ☞ Serving size= 10 tbsp, 150 g; GI= 15 (Low); GL= 2 (Low); Net carb= 14 g

Hummus (Homemade) ☞ Serving size= 10 tbsp, 150 g; GI= 15 (Low); GL= 4 (Low); Net carb= 24 g

Kidney Beans ☞ Serving size= ½ cup, 150 g; GI= 33 (Low); GL= 8.1 (Low); Net carb= 24.6 g

Kidney Beans—California Red Mature Seeds Cooked ☞ Serving size= ½ cup, 150 g; GI= 34 (Low); GL= 6.7 (Low); Net carb= 19.7 g

Kidney Beans—Red Mature Seeds Cooked ☞ Serving size= ½ cup, 150 g; GI= 33 (Low); GL= 7.6 (Low); Net carb= 23.1 g

Kidney Beans—Royal Red Mature Seeds Cooked ☞ Serving size= ½ cup, 150 g; GI= 33 (Low); GL= 6.2 (Low); Net carb= 18.8 g

Lentils (Cooked) ☞ Serving size= ½ cup, 150 g; GI= 21 (Low); GL= 3.9 (Low); Net carb= 18.3 g

Lentils—Dry Cooked ☞ Serving size= ½ cup, 150 g; GI= 21 (Low); GL= 3.8 (Low); Net carb= 18.2 g

Lentils—Mature Seeds Cooked ☞ Serving size= ½ cup, 150 g; GI= 21 (Low); GL= 3.7 (Low); Net carb= 17.5 g

Lima Beans ☞ Serving size= ½ cup, 150 g; GI= 46 (Low); GL= 9.6 (Low); Net carb= 20.8 g

Lima Beans—Dry Cooked ☛ Serving size= ½ cup, 150 g; GI= 46 (Low); GL= 9.5 (Low); Net carb= 20.7 g

Miso ☛ Serving size= 1 tbsp, 17 g; GI= 63 (Medium); GL= 2.1 (Low); Net carb= 3.4 g

Mung Beans—Dry Cooked ☛ Serving size= ½ cup, 150 g; GI= 42 (Low); GL= 7.2 (Low); Net carb= 17.2 g

Mung Beans—Mature Seeds Cooked ☛ Serving size= ½ cup, 150 g; GI= 42 (Low); GL= 7.3 (Low); Net carb= 17.3 g

Natto ☛ Serving size= ½ cup, 150 g; GI= 54 (Low); GL= 5.9 (Low); Net carb= 10.9 g

Navy Beans ☛ Serving size= ½ cup, 150 g; GI= 39 (Low); GL= 9.1 (Low); Net carb= 23.3 g

Navy Beans—Mature Seeds Cooked ☛ Serving size= ½ cup, 150 g; GI= 39 (Low); GL= 9.1 (Low); Net carb= 23.3 g

Okara ☛ Serving size= 1 cup, 122 g; GI= 53 (Low); GL= 7.9 (Low); Net carb= 14.9 g

Peanut Butter (Chunk Style) ☛ Serving size= 2 tbsp, 32 g; GI= 14 (Low); GL= 0.6 (Low); Net carb= 4.3 g

Peanut Butter (Smooth) ☛ Serving size= 2 tbsp, 32 g; GI= 14 (Low); GL= 0.8 (Low); Net carb= 5.8 g

Peanut Spread Reduced Sugar ☛ Serving size= 2 tbsp, 31 g; GI= 14 (Low); GL= 0.3 (Low); Net carb= 2 g

Peanuts—Spanish Raw ☛ Serving size= 1 cup, 146 g; GI= 13 (Low); GL= 1.2 (Low); Net carb= 9.2 g

Peanuts—Valencia Raw ☛ Serving size= 1 cup, 146 g; GI= 13 (Low); GL= 2.3 (Low); Net carb= 17.8 g

Peas—Dry Cooked ☛ Serving size= ½ cup, 150 g; GI= 22 (Low); GL= 3.5 (Low); Net carb= 16 g

Peas—Split Mature Seeds Cooked ☞ Serving size= ½ cup, 150 g; GI= 51 (Low); GL= 9.3 (Low); Net carb= 18.3 g

Pigeon Peas—Mature Seeds Cooked ☞ Serving size= ½ cup, 150 g; GI= 31 (Low); GL= 7.7 (Low); Net carb= 24.8 g

Pinto Beans—Canned Drained Solids ☞ Serving size= ½ cup, 150 g; GI= 39 (Low); GL= 8.6 (Low); Net carb= 22.1 g

Red Kidney Beans—Canned Drained , Cooked ☞ Serving size= ½ cup, 150 g; GI= 35 (Low); GL= 8.8 (Low); Net carb= 25.1 g

Red Kidney Beans—Dry Cooked ☞ Serving size= ½ cup, 150 g; GI= 35 (Low); GL= 8 (Low); Net carb= 22.9 g

Small White Beans—Mature Seeds Cooked ☞ Serving size= ½ cup, 150 g; GI= 36 (Low); GL= 8.3 (Low); Net carb= 23.1 g

Soft Tofu ☞ Serving size= 1 piece, 120 g; GI= 15 (Low); GL= 0.2 (Low); Net carb= 1.2 g

Soy Flour—Defatted ☞ Serving size= 1 cup, 105 g; GI= 25 (Low); GL= 4.3 (Low); Net carb= 17.2 g

Soy Flour—Full-Fat Raw ☞ Serving size= 1 cup, stirred, 84 g; GI= 25 (Low); GL= 4.7 (Low); Net carb= 18.7 g

Soy Flour—Full-Fat Roasted ☞ Serving size= 1 cup, stirred, 85 g; GI= 25 (Low); GL= 4.4 (Low); Net carb= 17.6 g

Soy Milk (All Flavors) Enhanced ☞ Serving size= 1 cup, 243 g; GI= 30 (Low); GL= 2.2 (Low); Net carb= 7.4 g

Soy Milk ☞ Serving size= 1 cup, 243 g; GI= 30 (Low); GL= 0.9 (Low); Net carb= 3 g

Soy Milk ☞ Serving size= 1 cup, 243 g; GI= 30 (Low); GL= 2.1 (Low); Net carb= 7 g

Soy Milk, Chai ☞ Serving size= 1 cup, 243 g; GI= 30 (Low); GL= 5.7 (Low); Net carb= 19 g

Soy Milk, Chocolate ☛ Serving size= 1 cup, 243 g; GI= 30 (Low); GL= 6.3 (Low); Net carb= 21.1 g

Soy Protein—Concentrate ☛ Serving size= 1 oz, 28.4 g; GI= 47 (Low); GL= 2.7 (Low); Net carb= 5.7 g

Soy Protein—Powder ☛ Serving size= 1 oz, 28.4 g; GI= 47 (Low); GL= 0 (Low); Net carb= 0 g

Soy Sauce without added sugar ☛ Serving size= 1 tbsp, 16 g; GI= 20 (Low); GL= 0.1 (Low); Net carb= 0.7 g

Soybean Curd ☛ Serving size= 1 slice, 29 g; GI= 15 (Low); GL= 0.3 (Low); Net carb= 2.3 g

Soybeans—Dry Cooked ☛ Serving size= 1 cup, 180 g; GI= 31 (Low); GL= 1.3 (Low); Net carb= 4.2 g

Soybeans—Mature Seeds Cooked ☛ Serving size= 1 cup, 172 g; GI= 31 (Low); GL= 1.3 (Low); Net carb= 4.1 g

Tamari, without added sugar ☛ Serving size= 1 tbsp, 18 g; GI= 20 (Low); GL= 0.2 (Low); Net carb= 0.9 g

Tempeh ☛ Serving size= 1 cup, 166 g; GI= 15 (Low); GL= 1.9 (Low); Net carb= 12.7 g

Tofu Silken Extra Firm ☛ Serving size= 1 slice, 84 g; GI= 15 (Low); GL= 0.2 (Low); Net carb= 1.6 g

Tofu Silken Firm ☛ Serving size= 1 slice, 84 g; GI= 15 (Low); GL= 0.3 (Low); Net carb= 1.9 g

White Beans—Mature Seeds Canned ☛ Serving size= ½ cup, 150 g; GI= 36 (Low); GL= 8.9 (Low); Net carb= 24.6 g

Yellow Beans—Mature Seeds Cooked ☛ Serving size= ½ cup, 150 g; GI= 36 (Low); GL= 8 (Low); Net carb= 22.3 g

# FISH & FISH PRODUCTS

Fish are part of the glycemic load eating pattern and provide high-quality proteins and good fats (Omega-3 and omega-6 fats) in addition to some key nutrients such as

• vitamin B2

• calcium and phosphorus

• iron

• iodine and choline

**The glycemic load of raw fish is equal to zero.**

Breading or battering fish should be avoided, especially when using simple carbohydrates such as white flour. Grilling, baking, broiling, poaching, or steaming fish is considered healthier since it does not rise the glycemic index of cooked fish.

---

Anchovy, canned, oil or water ☛ Serving size= 3 0z (85 g); GI= 0 (Low); GL= 0 (Low)

Anchovy, cooked, without flour ☞ Serving size= 3 0z (85 g); GI= 0 (Low); GL= 0 (Low)

Carp, floured, breaded or battered AND baked or fried ☞ Serving size= 3 0z (85 g); GI= 95 (High); GL= 7.8 (Low)

Carp, steamed or poached ☞ Serving size= 3 0z (85 g); GI= 0 (Low); GL= 0 (Low)

Catfish, floured, breaded or battered AND baked or fried ☞ Serving size= 1 fillet (150 g); GI= 95 (High); GL= 7.8 (Low)

Cod, floured, breaded or battered AND baked or fried, baked ☞ Serving size= 3 0z (85 g); GI= 95 (High); GL= 7.8 (Low)

Cod, floured, breaded or battered AND baked or fried, baked ☞ Serving size= 3 0z (85 g); GI= 95 (High); GL= 7.8 (Low)

Crab, cooked, without flour ☞ Serving size= 3 0z (85 g); GI= 0 (Low); GL= 0 (Low)

Crab, hard shell, steamed ☞ Serving size= 3 0z (85 g); GI= 0 (Low); GL= 0 (Low)

Crayfish, floured, breaded or battered AND baked or fried, baked ☞ Serving size= 3 0z (85 g); GI= 95 (High); GL= 7.8 (Low)

Croaker, floured or breaded, fried ☞ Serving size= 3 0z (85 g); GI= 95 (High); GL= 7.8 (Low)

Fish, in general, floured, breaded or battered AND baked or fried, baked ☞ Serving size= 3 0z (85 g); GI= 95 (High); GL= 7.8 (Low)

Fish, in general, canned, smoked, poached or steamed ☞ Serving size= 3 0z (85 g); GI= 0 (Low); GL= 0 (Low)

Flounder, floured, breaded or battered AND baked or fried, baked ☞ Serving size= 3 0z (85 g); GI= 95 (High); GL= 7.8 (Low)

Haddock, floured, breaded or battered AND baked or fried, baked ☞ Serving size= 3 0z (85 g); GI= 95 (High); GL= 7.8 (Low)

Haddock, floured, breaded or battered AND baked or fried ☞ Serving size= 3 0z (85 g); GI= 95 (High); GL= 7.8 (Low)

Mackerel, baked or broiled ☞ Serving size= 3 0z (85 g); GI= 0 (Low); GL= 1 (Low)

Mackerel, canned, smoked, poached or steamed ☞ Serving size= 3 0z (85 g); GI= 0 (Low); GL= 0 (Low)

Mackerel, floured, breaded or battered AND baked or fried, baked ☞ Serving size= 3 0z (85 g); GI= 95 (High); GL= 7.8 (Low)

Mullet, floured, breaded or battered AND baked or fried, baked ☞ Serving size= 1 fillet (150 g); GI= 95 (High); GL= 7.8 (Low)

Ocean perch, floured, breaded or battered AND baked or fried, baked ☞ Serving size= 1 fillet (150 g); GI= 95 (High); GL= 7.8 (Low)

Ocean perch, raw, steamed poached, baked or broiled ☞ Serving size= 1 fillet (150 g); GI= 0 (Low); GL= 0 (Low)

Perch, floured, breaded or battered AND baked or fried, baked ☞ Serving size= 1 fillet (150 g); GI= 95 (High); GL= 7.8 (Low)

Pompano, floured, breaded or battered AND baked or fried, baked ☞ Serving size= 1 fillet (150 g); GI= 95 (High); GL= 7.8 (Low)

Porgy, floured, breaded or battered AND baked or fried, baked ☞ Serving size= 1 fillet (150 g); GI= 95 (High); GL= 7.8 (Low)

Porgy, floured, breaded or battered AND baked or fried, baked ☞ Serving size= 1 fillet (150 g); GI= 95 (High); GL= 7.8 (Low)

Salmon, canned, smoked, poached or steamed ☞ Serving size= 1 fillet (150 g); GI= 0 (Low); GL= 0 (Low)

Salmon, floured or breaded, fried ☞ Serving size= 1 fillet (150 g); GI= 95 (High); GL= 7.8 (Low)

Sardines, canned in oil ☞ Serving size= 3 0z (85 g); GI= 0 (Low); GL= 0 (Low)

Sardines, cooked, without flour ☞ Serving size= 6 0z (170 g); GI= 0 (Low); GL= 0 (Low)

Sea bass, steamed poached, baked or broiled ☞ Serving size= 1 fillet (150 g); GI= 0 (Low); GL= 1 (Low)

Sea bass, floured, breaded or battered AND baked or fried, baked ☞ Serving size= 1 fillet (150 g); GI= 95 (High); GL= 8.2 (Low)

Shark, steamed poached, baked or broiled ☞ Serving size= 6 0z (170 g); GI= 0 (Low); GL= 0 (Low)

Shrimp, floured, fried ☞ Serving size= 3 0z (85 g); GI= 95 (High); GL= 8.2 (Low)

Smelt, floured, breaded or battered AND baked or fried, baked ☞ Serving size= 6 0z (170 g); GI= 95 (High); GL= 7.8 (Low)

Squid, breaded, fried ☞ Serving size= 6 0z (170 g); GI= 95 (High); GL= 7.8 (Low)

Swordfish, steamed poached, baked or broiled ☞ Serving size= 6 0z (170 g); GI= 0 (Low); GL= 1 (Low)

Swordfish, floured or breaded, fried ☞ Serving size= 6 0z (170 g); GI= 95 (High); GL= 7.8 (Low)

Swordfish, steamed poached, baked or broiled ☞ Serving size= 6 0z (170 g); GI= 0 (Low); GL= 1 (Low)

Trout, steamed poached, baked or broiled ☞ Serving size= 1 fillet (150 g); GI= 0 (Low); GL= 1 (Low)

Trout, floured, breaded or battered AND baked or fried, baked ☞ Serving size= 1 fillet (150 g); GI= 95 (High); GL= 7.8 (Low)

Trout, canned or smoked ☞ Serving size= 1 oz; GI= 0 (Low); GL= 0 (Low)

Tuna, canned, smoked, poached or steamed ☞ Serving size= 3 0z (85 g); GI= 0 (Low); GL= 0 (Low)

Tuna, fresh, baked or broiled ☞ Serving size= 6 0z (170 g); GI= 0 (Low); GL= 1 (Low)

Tuna, fresh, floured or breaded, fried ☞ Serving size= 6 0z (170 g); GI= 95 (High); GL= 7.8 (Low)

Whiting, steamed poached, baked or broiled ☞ Serving size= 6 0z (170 g); GI= 0 (Low); GL= 1 (Low)

Whiting, floured, breaded or battered AND baked or fried, baked ☞ Serving size= 6 0z (170 g); GI= 95 (High); GL= 7.8 (Low)

# FRUITS AND FRUITS PRODUCTS

Apple Baked, unsweetened ☛ Serving size= 1 apple with liquid, 161 (g); GI= 38 (Low); GL= 7.5 (Low); Net carbs= 19.7 g

Apple Chips ☛ Serving size= 1 cup, 28 (g); GI= 35 (Low); GL= 6.3 (Low); Net carbs= 17.9 g

Apple Pickled ☛ Serving size= 1 apple, 29 (g); GI= 38 (Low); GL= 3.4 (Low); Net carbs= 8.8 g

Apple Rings Fried ☛ Serving size= 1 ring, 19 (g); GI= 38 (Low); GL= 1.2 (Low); Net carbs= 3.2 g

Apples ☛ Serving size= 1 cup, quartered or chopped, 125 (g); GI= 38 (Low); GL= 5.4 (Low); Net carbs= 14.3 g

Apples, (Without Skin) ☛ Serving size= 1 cup slices, 110 (g); GI= 41 (Low); GL= 5.2 (Low); Net carbs= 12.6 g

Applesauce, Canned, unsweetened ☛ Serving size= 1 cup, 244 (g); GI= 38 (Low); GL= 9.4 (Low); Net carbs= 24.8 g

Apricots ☛ Serving size= 1 cup, halves, 155 (g); GI= 31 (Low); GL= 4.4 (Low); Net carbs= 14.1 g

Apricot Dried Cooked Without Sugar ☞ Serving size= 1/4 cup, 67.5 (g); GI= 41 (Low); GL= 7.8 (High); Net carbs= 19 g

Asian Pears ☞ Serving size= 1 fruit, 122 (g); GI= 26 (Low); GL= 2.2 (Low); Net carbs= 8.6 g

Avocados ☞ Serving size= 1 cup, cubes, 150 (g); GI= 50 (Low); GL= 1.4 (Low); Net carbs= 2.7 g

Banana, Ripe Fried ☞ Serving size= 1 small, 73 (g); GI= 62 (Medium); GL= 9.6 (Low); Net carbs= 15.5 g

Bartlett Pears ☞ Serving size= 1 cup, sliced, 140 (g); GI= 41 (Low); GL= 6.8 (Low); Net carbs= 16.7 g

Blackberries ☞ Serving size= 1 cup, 144 (g); GI= 25 (Low); GL= 1.6 (Low); Net carbs= 6.2 g

Blueberries raw or frozen ☞ Serving size= 1 cup, 148 (g); GI= 53 (Low); GL= 9.5 (Low); Net carbs= 17.9 g

Bosc Pear ☞ Serving size= 1 cup, sliced, 140 (g); GI= 41 (Low); GL= 7.5 (Low); Net carbs= 18.2 g

Boysenberries raw or Frozen ☞ Serving size= 1 cup, unthawed, 132 (g); GI= 43 (Low); GL= 3.9 (Low); Net carbs= 9.1 g

California Avocados ☞ Serving size= 1 cup, pureed, 230 (g); GI= 50 (Low); GL= 2.1 (Low); Net carbs= 4.2 g

California Grapefruit ☞ Serving size= 1 cup sections, with juice, 230 (g); GI= 25 (Low); GL= 5.6 (Low); Net carbs= 22.3 g

California Valencia Oranges ☞ Serving size= 1 cup sections, without membranes, 180 (g); GI= 42 (Low); GL= 7.1 (Low); Net carbs= 16.9 g

Cantaloupe Melons ☞ Serving size= 1 cup, balls, 177 (g); GI= 61 (Medium); GL= 7.8 (Low); Net carbs= 12.9 g

Casaba Melon ☞ Serving size= 1 cup, cubes, 170 (g); GI= 62 (Medium); GL= 6 (Low); Net carbs= 9.7 g

Cherries (Sweet) ☛ Serving size= 1 cup, with pits, yields, 138 (g); GI= 22 (Low); GL= 4.2 (Low); Net carbs= 19.2 g

Clementines ☛ Serving size= 1 fruit, 74 (g); GI= 35 (Low); GL= 2.7 (Low); Net carbs= 7.6 g

Cranberries ☛ Serving size= 1 cup, chopped, 110 (g); GI= 45 (Low); GL= 4.1 (Low); Net carbs= 9.2 g

Dates, Deglet Noor ☛ Serving size= 1/5 cup, chopped, 30 (g); GI= 44 (Low); GL= 8.7 (Low); Net carbs= 19.6 g

Dried Litchis ☛ Serving size= 1 fruit, 2.5 (g); GI= 60 (Medium); GL= 1 (Low); Net carbs= 1.7 g

European Black Currants ☛ Serving size= 1 cup, 112 (g); GI= 22 (Low); GL= 3.8 (Low); Net carbs= 17.2 g

Figs ☛ Serving size= 1 large, 64 (g); GI= 51 (Low); GL= 5.3 (Low); Net carbs= 10.4 g

Avocados ☛ Serving size= 1 cup, pureed, 230 (g); GI= 50 (Low); GL= 2.6 (Low); Net carbs= 5.1 g

Grapefruit ☛ Serving size= 1 cup sections, with juice, 230 (g); GI= 25 (Low); GL= 3.7 (Low); Net carbs= 14.7 g

Oranges ☛ Serving size= 1 cup sections, without membranes, 185 (g); GI= 42 (Low); GL= 7.1 (Low); Net carbs= 16.9 g

Fruit Salad, Fresh Or Raw Including Citrus Fruits No Dressing ☛ Serving size= 1 cup, 175 (g); GI= 51 (Low); GL= 10 (Low); Net carbs= 19.7 g

Fuji Apples ☛ Serving size= 1 cup, sliced, 109 (g); GI= 36 (Low); GL= 5.1 (Low); Net carbs= 14.3 g

Gala Apples ☛ Serving size= 1 cup, sliced, 109 (g); GI= 39 (Low); GL= 4.8 (Low); Net carbs= 12.4 g

Golden Delicious Apples ☛ Serving size= 1 cup, sliced, 109 (g); GI=

39 (Low); GL= 4.8 (Low); Net carbs= 12.2 g

Gooseberries ☛ Serving size= 1 cup, 150 (g); GI= 21 (Low); GL= 1.9 (Low); Net carbs= 8.8 g

Granny Smith Apples ☛ Serving size= 1 cup, sliced, 109 (g); GI= 36 (Low); GL= 4.2 (Low); Net carbs= 11.8 g

Grapefruit ☛ Serving size= 1 cup sections, with juice, 230 (g); GI= 25 (Low); GL= 4 (Low); Net carbs= 16.1 g

Grapes ☛ Serving size= 1 cup, 92 (g); GI= 53 (Low); GL= 7.9 (Low); Net carbs= 15 g

Green Olives Marinated ☛ Serving size= 1 olive, 2.7 (g); GI= 17 (Low); GL= 0 (Low); Net carbs= 0 g

Groundcherries ☛ Serving size= 1 cup, 140 (g); GI= 35 (Low); GL= 5.5 (Low); Net carbs= 15.7 g

Guavas ☛ Serving size= 1 cup, 165 (g); GI= 24 (Low); GL= 3.5 (Low); Net carbs= 14.7 g

Honeydew Melon ☛ Serving size= 1 cup, diced, 170 (g); GI= 62 (Medium); GL= 8.7 (Low); Net carbs= 14.1 g

Java Plum ☛ Serving size= 1 cup, 135 (g); GI= 25 (Low); GL= 5.3 (Low); Net carbs= 21 g

Kumquats ☛ Serving size= 1 fruit without refuse, 19 (g); GI= 0 (Low); GL= 0 (Low); Net carbs= 1.8 g

Lemon Juice, Raw ☛ Serving size= 1 cup, 244 (g); GI= 51 (Low); GL= 8.2 (Low); Net carbs= 16.1 g

Lime Juice ☛ Serving size= 1 cup, 242 (g); GI= 51 (Low); GL= 9.9 (Low); Net carbs= 19.4 g

Limes ☛ Serving size= 1 fruit, 67 (g); GI= 25 (Low); GL= 1.3 (Low); Net carbs= 5.2 g

Lychee, Canned in Syrup, Drained ☛ Serving size= 1 lychee with liquid, 21 (g); GI= 74 (High); GL= 3.6 (Low); Net carbs= 4.9 g

Mango Pickled ☞ Serving size= 1 slice, 28 (g); GI= 51 (Low); GL= 4.5 (Low); Net carbs= 8.9 g

Maraschino Cherries, Canned in Syrup, Drained ☞ Serving size= 1 cherry (nlea serving), 5 (g); GI= 85 (High); GL= 1.6 (Low); Net carbs= 1.9 g

Medjool Dates ☞ Serving size= 1 date, pitted, 24 (g); GI= 44 (Low); GL= 7.2 (Low); Net carbs= 16.4 g

Melon Balls ☞ Serving size= 1 cup, unthawed, 173 (g); GI= 62 (Medium); GL= 7.8 (Low); Net carbs= 12.5 g

Mulberries ☞ Serving size= 1 cup, 140 (g); GI= (); GL= 0 (Low); Net carbs= 11.3 g

Mushrooms Pickled ☞ Serving size= 1 cup, 156 (g); GI= (); GL= 0 (Low); Net carbs= 3.1 g

Nance, Canned in Syrup, Drained ☞ Serving size= 3 fruit without pits, 11.1 (g); GI= 85 (High); GL= 1.5 (Low); Net carbs= 1.8 g

Navel Oranges ☞ Serving size= 1 cup sections, without membranes, 165 (g); GI= 43 (Low); GL= 7.3 (Low); Net carbs= 17.1 g

Nectarines ☞ Serving size= 1 cup slices, 143 (g); GI= 35 (Low); GL= 4.4 (Low); Net carbs= 12.7 g

Olives ☞ Serving size= 1 tbsp, 8.4 (g); GI= 15 (Low); GL= 0.1 (Low); Net carbs= 0.4 g

Olives Black ☞ Serving size= 1 slice, 1 (g); GI= 15 (Low); GL= 0 (Low); Net carbs= 0 g

Olives Green Stuffed ☞ Serving size= 1 cup, 147 (g); GI= 15 (Low); GL= 0.2 (Low); Net carbs= 1.4 g

Oranges ☞ Serving size= 1 cup, sections, 180 (g); GI= 45 (Low); GL= 7.6 (Low); Net carbs= 16.8 g

Oranges Raw With Peel ☞ Serving size= 1 cup, 170 (g); GI= 45 (Low); GL= 8.4 (Low); Net carbs= 18.7 g

Papaya ☞ Serving size= 1 cup 1 inch pieces, 145 (g); GI= 60 (Medium); GL= 7.9 (Low); Net carbs= 13.2 g

Passion Fruit (Granadilla) ☞ Serving size= 1 cup, 236 (g); GI= 30 (Low); GL= 9.2 (Low); Net carbs= 30.6 g

Peach Pickled ☞ Serving size= 1 fruit, 88 (g); GI≈ 40 (Low); GL= 9.9 (Low); Net carbs= 24.8 g

Pears ☞ Serving size= 1 cup, slices, 140 (g); GI= 33 (Low); GL= 5.6 (Low); Net carbs= 17 g

Persimmons Native Raw ☞ Serving size= 1 fruit without refuse, 25 (g); GI= 61 (Medium); GL= 5.1 (Low); Net carbs= 8.4 g

Plum Pickled ☞ Serving size= 1 plum, 28 (g); GI= 24 (Low); GL= 2 (Low); Net carbs= 8.3 g

Plums ☞ Serving size= 1 cup, sliced, 165 (g); GI= 24 (Low); GL= 4 (Low); Net carbs= 16.5 g

Pomegranates ☞ Serving size= 1/2 cup arils (seed/juice sacs), 87 (g); GI= 53 (Low); GL= 6.8 (Low); Net carbs= 12.8 g

Prune Puree ☞ Serving size= 2 tbsp, 36 (g); GI= 43 (Low); GL= 9.6 (Low); Net carbs= 22.2 g

Pummelo ☞ Serving size= 1 cup, sections, 190 (g); GI= 22 (Low); GL= 3.6 (Low); Net carbs= 16.4 g

Quinces ☞ Serving size= 1 fruit without refuse, 92 (g); GI= 35 (Low); GL= 4.3 (Low); Net carbs= 12.3 g

Raspberries ☞ Serving size= 1 cup, 123 (g); GI= 78 (High); GL= 5.2 (Low); Net carbs= 6.7 g

Raspberries Cooked Or Canned unsweetened ☞ Serving size= 1 cup, 243 (g); GI= 77 (High); GL= 6.7 (Low); Net carbs= 8.7 g

Red And White Currants ☞ Serving size= 1 cup, 112 (g); GI= 25 (Low); GL= 2.7 (Low); Net carbs= 10.6 g

Red Delicious Apples ☞ Serving size= 1 cup, sliced, 109 (g); GI= 39 (Low); GL= 5 (Low); Net carbs= 12.8 g

Rhubarb ☞ Serving size= 1 cup, diced, 122 (g); GI= 15 (Low); GL= 0.5 (Low); Net carbs= 3.3 g

Sour Red Cherries ☞ Serving size= 1 cup, without pits, 155 (g); GI= 22 (Low); GL= 3.6 (Low); Net carbs= 16.4 g

Starfruit (Carambola) ☞ Serving size= 1 cup, cubes, 132 (g); GI= 45 (Low); GL= 2.3 (Low); Net carbs= 5.2 g

Strawberries ☞ Serving size= 1 cup, halves, 152 (g); GI= 41 (Low); GL= 3.5 (Low); Net carbs= 8.6 g

Tangerines Juices Canned ☞ Serving size= 1 cup, 189 (g); GI= 59 (Medium); GL= 9.2 (Low); Net carbs= 15.5 g

Watermelon ☞ Serving size= 1 cup, balls, 154 (g); GI= 72 (High); GL= 7.9 (Low); Net carbs= 11 g

# GRAINS AND PASTA

Barley Cooked ☞ Serving size= 1 cup (170 g); GI= 25 (Low); GL= 10 (Low); Net carb= 40 g

Bulgur, Cooked ☞ Serving size= 1 cup (140 g); GI= 47 (Low); GL= 8.6 (Low); Net carb= 18.4 g

Chinese Chow Mein Noodles ☞ Serving size= 1/2 cup dry (28 g); GI= 35 (Low); GL= 5.6 (Low); Net carb= 15.9 g

Corn Bran Crude ☞ Serving size= 1 cup (76 g); GI= 75 (High); GL= 3.8 (Low); Net carb= 5 g

Hominy Canned Yellow ☞ Serving size= 1 cup (160 g); GI= 40 (Low); GL= 7.5 (Low); Net carb= 18.8 g

Japanese Somen Cooked ☞ Serving size= 2 oz (57 g); GI= 41 (Low); GL= 6.4 (Low); Net carb= 15.7 g

Noodles Cooked, made with Rice ☞ Serving size= 2 oz (57 g); GI= 56 (Medium); GL= 7.3 (Low); Net carb= 13.1 g

Pasta Cooked, Homemade, Prepared With Egg ☞ Serving size= 2 oz (57 g); GI= 66 (Medium); GL= 8.9 (Low); Net carb= 13.4 g

Pasta Cooked, Homemade, Prepared without Egg ☛ Serving size= 2 oz (57 g); GI= 66 (Medium); GL= 9.5 (Low); Net carb= 14.3 g

Pearled Barley Cooked ☛ Serving size= 1 cup (157 g); GI= 25 (Low); GL= 9.6 (Low); Net carb= 38.3 g

Spaghetti Cooked, Spinach ☛ Serving size= 2 oz (57 g); GI= 33 (Low); GL= 4.9 (Low); Net carb= 14.9 g

# HERBS AND SPICES

Allspice ☞ Serving size= 1 tsp (2.1 g); GI= 15 (Low); GL= 0.3 (Low)

Anise seeds ☞ Serving size= 1 tsp (2.1 g); GI= 0.0 (Low); GL= 0.3 (Low)

Asian chives ☞ Serving size= 1 tbsp (3 g); GI= 15 (Low); GL= 0.3 (Low)

Basil ☞ Serving size= 1 tsp (0.7 g); GI= 70 (High); GL= 0 (Low)

Bay leaves ☞ Serving size= 1 tbsp, crumbled (1.8 g); GI= 23 (Low); GL= 0.1 (Low)

Black cumin ☞ Serving size= 1 tsp (2.4 g) ; GI= 0.0 (Low); GL= 0.3 (Low)

Black pepper ☞ Serving size= 1 tsp (2.4 g); GI= 44 (Low); GL= 0.3 (Low)

capers ☞ Serving size= 1 tbsp (8.6 g); GI= 20 (Low); GL= 1.4 (Low)

Caraway ☞ Serving size= 1 tbsp (6.7 g); GI= 5 (Low); GL= 1.1 (Low)

Cardamom ☛ Serving size= 1 tbsp (5.8 g); GI= 82 (High); GL= 1 (Low)

Cayenne pepper

☛ Serving size= 1 tsp (2.4 g); GI= 32 (Low); GL= 0.4 (Low)

Celery seed ☛ Serving size= 1 tbsp (5.8 g); GI= 32 (Low); GL= 0.9 (Low)

Chiles ☛ Serving size= 1 tbsp (8 g); GI= 42 (Low); GL= 1.3 (Low)

chilli ☛ Serving size= 1 tbsp (8 g); GI= 15 (Low); GL= 1.3 (Low)

Chives ☛ Serving size= 1 tbsp (2.8 g); GI= 15 (Low); GL= 0.3 (Low)

Cilantro

☛ Serving size= 1 cup (16 g); GI= 32 (Low); GL= 0 (Low)

Cinnamon ☛ Serving size= 1 tbsp (7.9 g); GI= 70 (High); GL= 2.1 (Low)

Cloves ☛ Serving size= 1 tbsp (6.6 g); GI= 87 (High); GL= 3.5 (Low)

Coriander seed ☛ Serving size= 1 tbsp (5 g); GI= 33 (Low); GL= 1 (Low)

Cumin ☛ Serving size= 1 tbsp (6 g); GI= 0.0 (Low); GL= 0 (Low)

Curry Leaves ☛ Serving size= 5 leaves (2g); GI= 5 (Low); GL= 0.1 (Low)

Curry powder ☛ Serving size= 1 tbsp (6 g); GI= 5 (Low); GL= 0.4 (Low)

Dill seed ☛ Serving size= 1 tsp (2.4 g); GI= 15 (Low); GL= 0.3 (Low)

Fennel seeds ☛ Serving size= 1 tbsp (5.8 g); GI= 16 (Low); GL= 0.3 (Low)

Fenugreek ☛ Serving size= 1 tbsp (11.1 g); GI= 25 (Low); GL= 0.6 (Low)

Fenugreek Leaves ☞ Serving size= 1 cup (85 g); GI= 25 (Low); GL= 0.6 (Low)

Five Spice Powder ☞ Serving size= 1 tsp (2.1 g) ; GI= 15 (Low); GL= 0.4 (Low)

Garlic chives ☞ Serving size= 2 clove (6 g); GI= 15 (Low); GL= 1 (Low)

Ginger ☞ Serving size= 1 tsp (2.1 g); GI= 72 (High); GL= 0.3 (Low)

Lemon Balm ☞ Serving size= 1 tsp (2.1 g); GI= 15 (Low); GL= 0.3 (Low)

Lemongrass ☞ Serving size= 1 cup (67 g); GI= 45 (Low); GL= 7.4 (Low)

Lime Leaves ☞ Serving size= 5 leaves (2 g); GI= 32 (Low); GL= 0.4 (Low)

Mint ☞ Serving size= 1 tbsp (3.1 g) ; GI= 10 (Low); GL= 0.2 (Low)

Mustard Seed ☞ Serving size= 1 tsp (2 g); GI= 32 (Low); GL= 0.2 (Low)

Nutmeg ☞ Serving size= 1 tsp (2.4 g); GI= 46 (Low); GL= 0.3 (Low)

Oregano ☞ Serving size= 1 tbsp (3 g); GI= 5 (Low); GL= 0.3 (Low)

Paprika ☞ Serving size= 1 tsp (2 g); GI= 15 (Low); GL= 0.3 (Low)

Parsley

☞ Serving size= 1 tbsp (3 g); GI= 32 (Low); GL= 0.3 (Low)

Poppy seeds ☞ Serving size= 1 tbsp (8.8 g); GI= 5 (Low); GL= 0.1 (Low)

Rosemary ☞ Serving size= 1 tbsp (3.3 g); GI= 70 (High); GL= 1.1 (Low)

Saffron ☞ Serving size= 1 tsp (0.7 g); GI= 70 (High); GL= 0.2 (Low)

Sage ☞ Serving size= 1 tsp (0.7 g); GI= 15 (Low); GL= 0.2 (Low)

Savory ☞ Serving size= 1 tbsp (4.4 g); GI= 16 (Low); GL= 0.2 (Low)

Sesame seeds ☞ Serving size= 1 tbsp (10 g); GI= 31 (Low); GL= 0.1 (Low)

Sumac ☞ Serving size= 1 tsp (2.7 g); GI= 43 (Low); GL= 0.2 (Low)

Summer Savoy ☞ Serving size= 1 tsp (2.7 g); GI= 21 (Low); GL= 0.2 (Low)

Tarragon ☞ Serving size= 1 tbsp (1.8g); GI= 15 (Low); GL= 0.1 (Low)

Thyme ☞ Serving size= 1 tbsp, leaves (2.7 g); GI= 51 (Low); GL= 0.1 (Low)

Turmeric ☞ Serving size= 1 tbsp (6.8 g); GI= 15 (Low); GL= 0.5 (Low)

Vanilla ☞ Serving size= 1 tbsp (4.4 g); GI= 16 (Low); GL= 0.5 (Low)

Wasabi powder ☞ Serving size= 1 tsp (2.8 g); GI= 31 (Low); GL= 0.3 (Low)

Watercress ☞ Serving size= 1 cup, chopped (34 g); GI= 32 (Low); GL= 0.1 (Low)

Wild garlic ☞ Serving size= 1 oz (28 g); GI= 11 (Low); GL= 2 (Low)

# VEGETABLES

Alfalfa sprouts, raw ☛ GI= 32 (Low); Serving size= 1 cup (33 g); GL= 0.3 (Low); Net carb= 0.2 g

Algae, dried ☛ GI= 32 (Low); Serving size= 1 serv (7 g); GL= 1 (Low); Net carb= 0 g

Artichoke— globe (French), cooked, from canned ☛ GI= 32 (Low); Serving size= 1 medium globe (103 g); GL= 1.4 (Low); Net carb= 4.5 g

Artichoke, globe (French), raw or cooked, from fresh or frozen or frozen ☛ GI= 32 (Low); Serving size= 1 medium globe (103 g); GL= 1.4 (Low); Net carb= 4.5 g

Artichoke— Jerusalem, raw ☛ GI= 32 (Low); Serving size= 1 whole artichoke (173 g); GL= 2.4 (Low); Net carb= 7.6 g

Artichoke— salad in oil ☛ GI= 32 (Low); Serving size= 1 medium globe (103 g); GL= 1.4 (Low); Net carb= 4.5 g

Asparagus— cooked, from canned ☛ GI= 32 (Low); Serving size= 8 spears (134 g); GL= 0.6 (Low); Net carb= 1.8 g

Asparagus, raw or cooked, from fresh or frozen ☛ GI= 32 (Low); Serving size= 8 spears (134 g); GL= 0.6 (Low); Net carb= 1.8 g

Asparagus— from canned, creamed or with cheese sauce ☛ GI= 28 (Low); Serving size= 8 spears (134 g); GL= 0.5 (Low); Net carb= 1.8 g

Asparagus— from fresh, creamed or with cheese sauce ☛ GI= 29 (Low); Serving size= 8 spears (134 g); GL= 0.5 (Low); Net carb= 1.8 g

Bean sprouts, raw or cooked, from fresh or frozen ☛ GI= 32 (Low); Serving size= 1 cup (129 g); GL= 1.7 (Low); Net carb= 5.4 g

Beet greens—raw ☛ GI= 32 (Low); Serving size= 1 cup (124 g); GL= 1.7 (Low); Net carb= 5.4 g

Beets— cooked, from canned ☛ GI= 64 (Medium); Serving size= 1 cup, canned (157 g); GL= 8.2 (Low); Net carb= 12.8 g

Beets, raw or cooked, from fresh or frozen ☛ GI= 64 (Medium); Serving size= 1 cup, diced (157 g); GL= 8.2 (Low); Net carb= 12.8 g

Beets— pickled ☛ GI= 66 (Medium); Serving size= 1 cup, diced (157 g); GL= 8.4 (Low); Net carb= 12.8 g

Beets— raw ☛ GI= 64 (Medium); Serving size= 1 cup, diced (157 g); GL= 8.2 (Low); Net carb= 12.8 g

Broccoflower, Cooked ☛ GI= 32 (Low); Serving size= 1 cup (87 g); GL= 0.8 (Low); Net carb= 2.6 g

Broccoli—raw ☛ GI= 32 (Low); Serving size= 1 medium stalk (148 g); GL= 1.9 (Low); Net carb= 5.9 g

Brussels sprouts—raw ☛ GI= 32 (Low); Serving size= 1 cup (160 g); GL= 2.3 (Low); Net carb= 7.2 g

Cabbage—Chinese, cooked or raw ☛ GI= 32 (Low); Serving size= 1 cup, shredded (170 g); GL= 0.4 (Low); Net carb= 1.4 g

Cabbage—fresh, pickled, Japanese style ☛ GI= 32 (Low); Serving size= 1 cup (150 g); GL= 1.2 (Low); Net carb= 3.9 g

Cabbage—green, cooked ☞ GI= 32 (Low); Serving size= 1 cup (150 g); GL= 1.7 (Low); Net carb= 5.3 g

Cabbage—green, raw ☞ GI= 32 (Low); Serving size= 1 cup (150 g); GL= 1.7 (Low); Net carb= 5.3 g

Cabbage—Kim Chee style ☞ GI= 32 (Low); Serving size= 1 cup (150 g); GL= 1.7 (Low); Net carb= 5.3 g

Cabbage—red, cooked ☞ GI= 32 (Low); Serving size= 1 cup (150 g); GL= 1.7 (Low); Net carb= 5.3 g

Cabbage—red, pickled or raw ☞ GI= 32 (Low); Serving size= 1 cup (150 g); GL= 1.7 (Low); Net carb= 5.3 g

Cactus—cooked ☞ GI= 7 (Low); Serving size= 1 cup (150 g); GL= 0.1 (Low); Net carb= 2 g

Cactus—raw ☞ GI= 7 (Low); Serving size= 1 cup (150 g); GL= 0.1 (Low); Net carb= 1.9 g

Calabaza (Spanish pumpkin), cooked ☞ GI= 75 (High); Serving size= 1 cup, cubes (166 g); GL= 6.2 (Low); Net carb= 8.3 g

Carrots, raw, cooked or canned ☞ GI= 47 (Low); Serving size= 1 cup or 1 carrot (151 g); GL= 4.8 (Low); Net carb= 10.2 g

Cauliflower, raw or pickled ☞ GI= 32 (Low); Serving size= 1 cup chopped (107 g); GL= 0.6 (Low); Net carb= 1.9 g

Celery juice ☞ GI= 32 (Low); Serving size= 1 cup (240 g); GL= 1.8 (Low); Net carb= 5.5 g

Celery, raw or cooked ☞ GI= 32 (Low); Serving size= 1 cup, diced (150 g); GL= 1.1 (Low); Net carb= 3.5 g

Chard, cooked ☞ GI= 32 (Low); Serving size= 1 cup, stalk and leaves (150 grams); GL= 1 (Low); Net carb= 3 g

Christophine—cooked ☞ GI= 32 (Low); Serving size= 1 cup (165 g); GL= 1.2 (Low); Net carb= 3.8 g

Coleslaw, with dressing ☛ GI= 44 (Low); Serving size= 1 cup (120 g); GL= 5.8 (Low); Net carb= 13.2 g

Collards, raw, or cooked, from fresh , frozen or canned ☛ GI= 32 (Low); Serving size= 1 cup, canned (170 g); GL= 2.3 (Low); Net carb= 7.3 g

Corn Cooked, From Fresh, Canned or Frozen ☛ GI= 48 (Low); Serving size= 1 cup (169 g); GL= 9.8 (Low); Net carb= 20.3 g

Corn Dried Cooked ☛ GI= 48 (Low); Serving size= 1 oz (28 g); GL= 1.8 (Low); Net carb= 3.8 g

Cucumber salad, prepared with oil, and vinegar ☛ GI= 32 (Low); Serving size= 1 cup (185 g); GL= 2.3 (Low); Net carb= 7.2 g

Cucumber salad, prepared with creamy dressing ☛ GI= 32 (Low); Serving size= 1 cup (185 g); GL= 2.3 (Low); Net carb= 7.2 g

Cucumber, raw or cooked ☛ GI= 32 (Low); Serving size= 1 cup (185 g); GL= 2.3 (Low); Net carb= 7.2 g

Cucumber, pickles, dill or fresh ☛ GI= 32 (Low); Serving size= 1 cup (185 g); GL= 2.3 (Low); Net carb= 7.2 g

Dandelion greens—raw ☛ GI= 32 (Low); Serving size= 1 cup (55 grams); GL= 0.6 (Low); Net carb= 1.9 g

Eggplant—cooked ☛ GI= 32 (Low); Serving size= 1 cup (99 g); GL= 1.8 (Low); Net carb= 5.6 g

Eggplant—pickled ☛ GI= 32 (Low); Serving size= 1 cup (155 g); GL= 2.8 (Low); Net carb= 8.7 g

Endive—raw ☛ GI= 32 (Low); Serving size= 1 cup, chopped (50 g); GL= 0.1 (Low); Net carb= 0.3 g

Fennel ☛ GI= 16 (Low); Serving size= 1 cup, sliced (87 g); GL= 0.6 (Low); Net carb= 3.7 g

Fennel Bulb—Cooked ☛ GI= 16 (Low); Serving size= 1 fennel bulb (218 g); GL= 2.3 (Low); Net carb= 14.1 g

Jicama—raw ☛ GI= 22 (Low); Serving size= 1 cup (130 g); GL= 1.5 (Low); Net carb= 6.6 g

Kale, raw ☛ GI= 32 (Low); Serving size= 1 cup 1 inch pieces (16 g); GL= 0 (Low); Net carb= 0.1 g

Kale, Cooked From Canned, Fresh or Frozen ☛ GI= 32 (Low); Serving size= 1 cup, chopped (130 g); GL= 1.2 (Low); Net carb= 3.9 g

Kohlrabi, raw ☛ GI= 21 (Low); Serving size= 1 cup (135 g); GL= 0.7 (Low); Net carb= 3.5 g

Kohlrabi, Cooked, Boiled Drained ☛ GI= 21 (Low); Serving size= 1 cup slices (165 g); GL= 1.9 (Low); Net carb= 9.2 g

Kohlrabi Creamed ☛ GI= 21 (Low); Serving size= 1 cup (187 g); GL= 2.8 (Low); Net carb= 13.2 g

Leeks, raw ☛ GI= 32 (Low); Serving size= 1 cup slices (165 g); GL= 6.5 (Low); Net carb= 20.4 g

Leeks, Cooked Bulb And Lower Leaf-Portion ☛ GI= 32 (Low); Serving size= 1 cup (170 g); GL= 3.6 (Low); Net carb= 11.3 g

Lettuce, arugula, raw ☛ GI= 32 (Low); Serving size= 1/6 medium head (89 g); GL= 0.7 (Low); Net carb= 2.3 g

Lettuce—Boston, raw ☛ GI= 32 (Low); Serving size= 1/6 medium head (89 g); GL= 0.7 (Low); Net carb= 2.3 g

Lettuce, raw or cooked ☛ GI= 32 (Low); Serving size= 1/6 medium head (89 g); GL= 0.7 (Low); Net carb= 2.3 g

Lotus Root, Cooked From Fresh, Frozen or Canned ☛ GI= 34 (Low); Serving size= 10 slices (81 g); GL= 3.4 (Low); Net carb= 10 g

Mushrooms, Cooked, From Canned, Fresh, or Frozen ☛ GI= 22 (Low); Serving size= 5 medium (89 g); GL= 0.5 (Low); Net carb= 2.3 g

Mushrooms, Creamed From Fresh, Frozen or Canned ☛ GI= 22 (Low); Serving size= 1 cup (217 g); GL= 2.6 (Low); Net carb= 11.9 g

Mushrooms Portobellos Grilled ☛ GI= 24 (Low); Serving size= 1 cup sliced (121 g); GL= 0.7 (Low); Net carb= 2.7 g

Mushrooms Shiitake, Cooked or Stir-Fried ☛ GI= 22 (Low); Serving size= 1 cup pieces (145 g); GL= 3.9 (Low); Net carb= 17.8 g

Mustard Cabbage, Cooked ☛ GI= 32 (Low); Serving size= 1 cup (175 g); GL= 0.4 (Low); Net carb= 1.3 g

Mustard Greens raw ☛ GI= 33 (Low); Serving size= 1 cup, chopped (56 g); GL= 0.3 (Low); Net carb= 0.8 g

Mustard Greens, Cooked From Fresh, Frozen or Canned ☛ GI= 33 (Low); Serving size= 1 cup, chopped (140 g); GL= 1.2 (Low); Net carb= 3.5 g

Mustard Spinach, raw ☛ GI= 32 (Low); Serving size= 1 cup, chopped (150 g); GL= 0.5 (Low); Net carb= 1.7 g

Mustard Spinach, Cooked ☛ GI= 32 (Low); Serving size= 1 cup, chopped (180 g); GL= 0.5 (Low); Net carb= 1.4 g

New Zealand Spinach ☛ GI= 33 (Low); Serving size= 1 cup, chopped (56 g); GL= 0.2 (Low); Net carb= 0.6 g

New Zealand Spinach, Cooked ☛ GI= 33 (Low); Serving size= 1 cup, chopped (180 g); GL= 0.4 (Low); Net carb= 1.3 g

Nopales ☛ GI= 35 (Low); Serving size= 1 cup, sliced (86 g); GL= 0.3 (Low); Net carb= 1 g

Okra ☛ GI= 32 (Low); Serving size= 1 cup (100 g); GL= 1.4 (Low); Net carb= 4.3 g

Okra Cooked, From Fresh, Frozen or Canned ☛ GI= 32 (Low); Serving size= 1/2 cup slices (80 g); GL= 0.5 (Low); Net carb= 1.6 g

Onions ☞ GI= 15 (Low); Serving size= 1 cup, chopped (160 g); GL= 1.8 (Low); Net carb= 12.2 g

Onions Cooked, From Fresh, Frozen or Canned ☞ GI= 15 (Low); Serving size= 1 onion (63 g); GL= 0.3 (Low); Net carb= 1.8 g

Onions Dehydrated Flakes ☞ GI= 18 (Low); Serving size= 1 tbsp (5 g); GL= 0.7 (Low); Net carb= 3.7 g

Onions Creamed, From Fresh or Frozen ☞ GI= 15 (Low); Serving size= 1 cup (228 g); GL= 3 (Low); Net carb= 20 g

Onions Pearl Cooked, From Fresh, Frozen or Canned ☞ GI= 15 (Low); Serving size= 1 cup (185 g); GL= 2.4 (Low); Net carb= 16.1 g

Oriental Radishes ☞ GI= 32 (Low); Serving size= 1 cup slices (116 g); GL= 1.2 (Low); Net carb= 3.7 g

Oyster Mushrooms ☞ GI= 24 (Low); Serving size= 1 large (148 g); GL= 1.5 (Low); Net carb= 6.4 g

Palm Hearts, Canned ☞ GI= 38 (Low); Serving size= 1 cup (146 g); GL= 1.2 (Low); Net carb= 3.2 g

Parsley ☞ GI= 32 (Low); Serving size= 1 cup chopped (60 g); GL= 0.6 (Low); Net carb= 1.8 g

Parsnips ☞ GI= 48 (Low); Serving size= 1 cup slices (133 g); GL= 8.4 (Low); Net carb= 17.4 g

Parsnips, Cooked ☞ GI= 48 (Low); Serving size= 1/2 cup slices (78 g); GL= 4.9 (Low); Net carb= 10.1 g

Peas, green cooked, From Fresh, Frozen or Canned ☞ GI= 48 (Low); Serving size= 1 cup (175 g); GL= 8.3 (Low); Net carb= 17.3 g

Peas, green—raw ☞ GI= 48 (Low); Serving size= 1 cup (175 g); GL= 8.3 (Low); Net carb= 17.3 g

Pepper—hot chili, raw ☞ GI= 32 (Low); Serving size= 1 pepper (73 g); GL= 0.9 (Low); Net carb= 2.8 g

Pepper hot cooked, from Fresh, Frozen or canned ☛ GI= 32 (Low); Serving size= 1 pepper (73 g); GL= 0.9 (Low); Net carb= 2.8 g

Pepper—hot, pickled ☛ GI= 32 (Low); Serving size= 1 pepper (73 g); GL= 0.9 (Low); Net carb= 2.8 g

Pepper—pickled ☛ GI= 32 (Low); Serving size= 1 pepper (73 g); GL= 0.9 (Low); Net carb= 2.8 g

Pepper—poblano, raw ☛ GI= 32 (Low); Serving size= 1 pepper (73 g); GL= 0.9 (Low); Net carb= 2.8 g

Pepper—Serrano, raw ☛ GI= 32 (Low); Serving size= 1 cup (110 g); GL= 4.2 (Low); Net carb= 13.2 g

Pepper—sweet, green, raw ☛ GI= 32 (Low); Serving size= 1 cup (110 g); GL= 4.1 (Low); Net carb= 12.9 g

Pepper—sweet, red, raw ☛ GI= 32 (Low); Serving size= 1 cup (110 g); GL= 4.2 (Low); Net carb= 13 g

Pigeon peas—cooked ☛ GI= 22 (Low); Serving size= 1 cup (125 g); GL= 3.6 (Low); Net carb= 16.3 g

Pimiento ☛ GI= 32 (Low); Serving size= 1 cup (185 g); GL= 4.7 (Low); Net carb= 14.8 g

Radish—common, raw ☛ GI= 32 (Low); Serving size= 1 cup slices (116 g); GL= 1.9 (Low); Net carb= 5.9 g

Radish—raw ☛ GI= 32 (Low); Serving size= 1 cup slices (116 g); GL= 1.2 (Low); Net carb= 3.7 g

Romaine Lettuce ☛ GI= 32 (Low); Serving size= 1 cup shredded (47 g); GL= 0.2 (Low); Net carb= 0.6 g

Rutabaga Cooked ☛ GI= 72 (High); Serving size= 1 cup, pieces (175 g); GL= 6.2 (Low); Net carb= 8.6 g

Salsify, Raw ☛ GI= 30 (Low); Serving size= 1 cup slices (133 g); GL= 6.1 (Low); Net carb= 20.3 g

Salsify Cooked, From Fresh, Frozen or Canned ☛ GI= 30 (Low); Serving size= 1 cup slices (135 g); GL= 5 (Low); Net carb= 16.6 g

Sauerkraut ☛ GI= 32 (Low); Serving size= 1 cup (142 g); GL= 0.6 (Low); Net carb= 2 g

Sauerkraut Cooked, From Fresh, Frozen or canned ☛ GI= 32 (Low); Serving size= 1 cup (142 g); GL= 0.7 (Low); Net carb= 2.1 g

Savoy Cabbage ☛ GI= 32 (Low); Serving size= 1 cup, shredded (70 g); GL= 0.7 (Low); Net carb= 2.1 g

Scallop Squash ☛ GI= 48 (Low); Serving size= 1 cup slices (130 g); GL= 1.6 (Low); Net carb= 3.4 g

Seaweed Agar Raw ☛ GI= 48 (Low); Serving size= 2 tbsp (1/8 cup) (10 g); GL= 0.3 (Low); Net carb= 0.6 g

Snow Peas Cooked, From Fresh, Frozen or Canned ☛ GI= 30 (Low); Serving size= 1 cup, chopped (98 g); GL= 1.5 (Low); Net carb= 4.9 g

Soybean Sprouts ☛ GI= 15 (Low); Serving size= 1/2 cup (35 g); GL= 0.4 (Low); Net carb= 3 g

Soybeans Green Cooked ☛ GI= 15 (Low); Serving size= 1 cup (180 g); GL= 1.8 (Low); Net carb= 12.3 g

Soybeans Mature Seeds Cooked ☛ GI= 15 (Low); Serving size= 1 cup (94 g); GL= 0.8 (Low); Net carb= 5.4 g

Spaghetti Squash ☛ GI= 20 (Low); Serving size= 1 cup, cubes (101 g); GL= 1.1 (Low); Net carb= 5.4 g

Spinach Cooked, From Fresh, Frozen or Canned ☛ GI= 18 (Low); Serving size= 1 cup (30 g); GL= 0.1 (Low); Net carb= 0.4 g

Spring Onions ☛ GI= 15 (Low); Serving size= 1 cup, chopped (100 g); GL= 0.7 (Low); Net carb= 4.7 g

Squash Spaghetti, Cooked ☛ GI= 20 (Low); Serving size= 1 cup, cooked, (160 g); GL= 1.5 (Low); Net carb= 7.7 g

Squash Summer ☞ GI= 15 (Low); Serving size= 1 cup (217 g); GL= 1.7 (Low); Net carb= 11.6 g

Squash Winter, Cooked ☞ GI= 15 (Low); Serving size= 1 cup, cubes (205 g); GL= 1.9 (Low); Net carb= 12.4 g

Sun-Dried Tomatoes ☞ GI= 36 (Low); Serving size= 1 cup (54 g); GL= 8.4 (Low); Net carb= 23.5 g

Swamp Cabbage ☞ GI= 32 (Low); Serving size= 1 cup, chopped (56 g); GL= 0.2 (Low); Net carb= 0.6 g

Swamp Cabbage Cooked ☞ GI= 32 (Low); Serving size= 1 cup, chopped (98 g); GL= 0.6 (Low); Net carb= 1.8 g

Sweet Potato Cooked, Boiled ☞ GI= 66 (Medium); Serving size= 1 small (80 g); GL= 7.6 (Low); Net carb= 11.5 g

Swiss Chard ☞ GI= 32 (Low); Serving size= 1 cup (36 g); GL= 0.2 (Low); Net carb= 0.8 g

Taro ☞ GI= 32 (Low); Serving size= 1 cup, sliced (104 g); GL= 7.4 (Low); Net carb= 23.3 g

Taro Leaves Cooked ☞ GI= 32 (Low); Serving size= 1 cup (145 g); GL= 0.9 (Low); Net carb= 2.7 g

Taro Leaves Raw ☞ GI= 32 (Low); Serving size= 1 cup (28 g); GL= 0.3 (Low); Net carb= 0.8 g

Tomatillos ☞ GI= 38 (Low); Serving size= 1 medium (34 g); GL= 0.5 (Low); Net carb= 1.3 g

Tomatoes ☞ GI= 38 (Low); Serving size= 1 cup cherry tomatoes (149 g); GL= 1.5 (Low); Net carb= 4 g

Tomatoes, Cooked, From Fresh, Frozen or Canned ☞ GI= 38 (Low); Serving size= 1 cup (240 g); GL= 3 (Low); Net carb= 7.9 g

Tomatoes Crushed Canned ☞ GI= 38 (Low); Serving size= 1/2 cup (121 g); GL= 2.5 (Low); Net carb= 6.5 g

Sun-Dried Tomatoes Packed In Oil ☛ GI= 38 (Low); Serving size= 1 cup (110 g); GL= 7.3 (Low); Net carb= 19.3 g

Turnip Cooked, From Fresh, Frozen or Canned ☛ GI= 32 (Low); Serving size= 1 cup, pieces (155 g); GL= 1.5 (Low); Net carb= 4.7 g

Turnip Greens ☛ GI= 32 (Low); Serving size= 1 cup, chopped (55 g); GL= 0.7 (Low); Net carb= 2.2 g

Wakame ☛ GI= 50 (Low); Serving size= 2 tbsp (1/8 cup) (10 g); GL= 0.4 (Low); Net carb= 0.9 g

Wasabi Root ☛ GI= 41 (Low); Serving size= 1 cup, sliced (130 g); GL= 8.4 (Low); Net carb= 20.5 g

Waterchestnuts Chinese Raw or Canned ☛ GI= 54 (Low); Serving size= 1/2 cup slices (62 g); GL= 7 (Low); Net carb= 13 g

Watercress ☛ GI= 32 (Low); Serving size= 1 cup, chopped (34 g); GL= 0.1 (Low); Net carb= 0.3 g

Watercress, Cooked ☛ GI= 32 (Low); Serving size= 1 cup (142 g); GL= 0.3 (Low); Net carb= 1 g

Winged Bean Immature Seeds, Cooked ☛ GI= 50 (Low); Serving size= 1 cup (62 g); GL= 1 (Low); Net carb= 2 g

Winged Beans Immature Seeds Raw ☛ GI= 50 (Low); Serving size= 1 cup slices (44 g); GL= 0.9 (Low); Net carb= 1.9 g

Winter Squash ☛ GI= 51 (Low); Serving size= 1 cup, cubes (116 g); GL= 4.2 (Low); Net carb= 8.2 g

Yardlong Bean Cooked ☛ GI= 82 (High); Serving size= 1 cup slices (104 g); GL= 7.8 (Low); Net carb= 9.5 g

Yardlong Bean Raw ☛ GI= 82 (High); Serving size= 1 cup slices (91 g); GL= 6.2 (Low); Net carb= 7.6 g

Zucchini ☛ GI= 15 (Low); Serving size= 1 cup, chopped (124 g); GL= 0.4 (Low); Net carb= 2.6 g

# PART VIII
# FOODS WITH MODERATE
# GLYCEMIC LOAD

# BAKED PRODUCTS

Baklava ☛ Serving size= 1 piece, 78 g; GI= 63 (Medium); GL= 17.1 (Medium); Net carb= 27.2 g

Bread, 100% Barley Flour ☛ Serving size= 1 slice, 1 oz, 28.4 g; GI= 67 (Medium); GL= 11.4 (Medium); Net carb= 17 g

Bread, Baguette French ☛ Serving size= 1 slice, 1 oz, 28.4 g; GI= 95 (High); GL= 13.2 (Medium); Net carb= 13.9 g

Bread, Cheese ☛ Serving size= 1 slice, 48 g; GI= 72 (High); GL= 14.8 (Medium); Net carb= 20.5 g

Bread, Cornmeal And Molasses ☛ Serving size= 1 slice, 1 oz, 28.4 g; GI= 81 (High); GL= 12.3 (Medium); Net carb= 15.2 g

Bread, Focaccia Plain ☛ Serving size= 1 piece, 57 g; GI= 70 (High); GL= 13.6 (Medium); Net carb= 19.4 g

Bread, Garlic (average) ☛ Serving size= 1 small slice, 39 g; GI= 81 (High); GL= 12.4 (Medium); Net carb= 15.3 g

Bread, Naan Indian Flatbread ☛ Serving size= 1 piece, 44 g; GI= 63 (Medium); GL= 12.5 (Medium); Net carb= 19.8 g

Bread, White Flour ☛ Serving size= 1 slice, 1 oz, 28.4 g; GI= 71 (High); GL= 14.1 (Medium); Net carb= 19.9 g

Cake Or Cupcake, Applesauce (average value) ☛ Serving size= 1 regular piece, 75 g; GI= 55 (Medium); GL= 18.8 (Medium); Net carb= 34.1 g

Cake Or Cupcake, Banana (average value) ☛ Serving size= 1 regular piece, 50 g; GI= 55 (Medium); GL= 12.8 (Medium); Net carb= 23.3 g

Cake Or Cupcake, Gingerbread ☛ Serving size= 1 regular piece, 50 g; GI= 55 (Medium); GL= 13.6 (Medium); Net carb= 24.7 g

Cake Or Cupcake, Lemon ☛ Serving size= 1 regular piece, 50 g; GI= 55 (Medium); GL= 12.4 (Medium); Net carb= 22.5 g

Cake Or Cupcake, Nut ☛ Serving size= 1 regular piece, 50 g; GI= 55 (Medium); GL= 12.3 (Medium); Net carb= 22.4 g

Cake Or Cupcake, Oatmeal ☛ Serving size= 1 regular piece, 50 g; GI= 55 (Medium); GL= 17 (Medium); Net carb= 30.9 g

Cake Or Cupcake, Peanut Butter ☛ Serving size= 1 regular piece, 50 g; GI= 55 (Medium); GL= 14.5 (Medium); Net carb= 26.4 g

Cake, FruitCake (Commercially Made) ☛ Serving size= 1 oz, 28.4 g; GI= 66 (Medium); GL= 10.8 (Medium); Net carb= 16.4 g

Cake, Sponge (Commercially Made) ☛ Serving size= 1 oz, 28.4 g; GI= 66 (Medium); GL= 11.4 (Medium); Net carb= 17.2 g

Coookie, Biscotti ☛ Serving size= 1 cookie, 32 g; GI= 69 (Medium); GL= 14.4 (Medium); Net carb= 20.9 g

Coookie, Brownie With Filling ☛ Serving size= 1 small, 40 g; GI= 69 (Medium); GL= 17.1 (Medium); Net carb= 24.8 g

Coookie, Chocolate Coating ☛ Serving size= 4 cookies, 32 g; GI= 69 (Medium); GL= 14.5 (Medium); Net carb= 21 g

Coookie, Lemon Bar ☛ Serving size= 4 cookies, 32 g; GI= 69 (Medium); GL= 13.6 (Medium); Net carb= 19.7 g

Crackers, Cheese Whole Grain ☛ Serving size= 1 serving 55 pieces, 31 g; GI= 65 (Medium); GL= 10.3 (Medium); Net carb= 15.8 g

Crackers, Meal ☛ Serving size= 1 oz, 28.4 g; GI= 65 (Medium); GL= 14.4 (Medium); Net carb= 22.2 g

Crackers, Wheat Regular ☛ Serving size= 16 crackers 1 serving, 34 g; GI= 70 (High); GL= 15.2 (Medium); Net carb= 21.7 g

Crackers, Whole-Wheat ☛ Serving size= 1 serving, 28 g; GI= 66 (Medium); GL= 11 (Medium); Net carb= 16.6 g

Doughnut Chocolate ☛ Serving size= 1 doughnut, 53 g; GI= 77 (High); GL= 18.6 (Medium); Net carb= 24.2 g

Doughnut, Chocolate, Sugared Or Glazed ☛ Serving size= 1 oz, 28.4 g; GI= 76 (High); GL= 11.9 (Medium); Net carb= 15.7 g

Doughnut, Cake-Type Plain Chocolate-Coated Or Frosted ☛ Serving size= 1 oz, 28.4 g; GI= 78 (High); GL= 10.9 (Medium); Net carb= 14 g

Doughnut, Plain Sugared Or Glazed ☛ Serving size= 1 oz, 28.4 g; GI= 79 (High); GL= 11.1 (Medium); Net carb= 14 g

Doughnut, Chocolate Raised Or Yeast ☛ Serving size= 1 doughnut, 50 g; GI= 77 (High); GL= 17.3 (Medium); Net carb= 22.5 g

Fig Bars ☛ Serving size= 1 oz, 28.4 g; GI= 78 (High); GL= 14.7 (Medium); Net carb= 18.8 g

Melba Toast ☛ Serving size= 1 slice, 1 oz, 28.4 g; GI= 70 (High); GL= 14 (Medium); Net carb= 20 g

Muffin, Carrot ☛ Serving size= 1 muffin, 58 g; GI= 59 (Medium); GL= 14.6 (Medium); Net carb= 24.8 g

Muffin, Chocolate ☛ Serving size= 1 muffin, 58 g; GI= 59 (Medium); GL= 16.8 (Medium); Net carb= 28.4 g

Muffin, English Cheese ☛ Serving size= 1 muffin, 58 g; GI= 59 (Medium); GL= 13.3 (Medium); Net carb= 22.5 g

Muffin, English Wheat Bran Raisins ☛ Serving size= 1 muffin, 58 g; GI= 70 (High); GL= 17.8 (Medium); Net carb= 25.4 g

Muffin, English With Fruit ☛ Serving size= 1 muffin, 58 g; GI= 70 (High); GL= 17.8 (Medium); Net carb= 25.4 g

Muffin, English With Raisins ☛ Serving size= 1 muffin, 58 g; GI= 70 (High); GL= 17.9 (Medium); Net carb= 25.6 g

Muffin, Oatmeal ☛ Serving size= 1 muffin, 58 g; GI= 53 (Low); GL= 13 (Medium); Net carb= 24.6 g

Muffin, Pumpkin ☛ Serving size= 1 muffin, 58 g; GI= 53 (Low); GL= 12.8 (Medium); Net carb= 24.2 g

Muffin, Wheat ☛ Serving size= 1 muffin, 58 g; GI= 55 (Medium); GL= 14 (Medium); Net carb= 25.5 g

Muffin, Wheat Bran ☛ Serving size= 1 muffin, 58 g; GI= 50 (Low); GL= 10.7 (Medium); Net carb= 21.3 g

Pie, Coconut Cream ☛ Serving size= 1 tart, 117 g; GI= 59 (Medium); GL= 17.1 (Medium); Net carb= 28.9 g

Pie, Custard ☛ Serving size= 1 tart, 117 g; GI= 59 (Medium); GL= 17.9 (Medium); Net carb= 30.4 g

Roll, Cheese ☛ Serving size= 1 roll, 41 g; GI= 73 (High); GL= 14.3 (Medium); Net carb= 19.6 g

Roll, Dinner Rye ☛ Serving size= 1 large , 43 g; GI= 77 (High); GL= 15.9 (Medium); Net carb= 20.7 g

Strudel, Berry ☛ Serving size= 1 piece, 64 g; GI= 59 (Medium); GL= 16.6 (Medium); Net carb= 28.1 g

Strudel, Cheese ☛ Serving size= 1 piece, 64 g; GI= 59 (Medium); GL= 13.9 (Medium); Net carb= 23.6 g

Strudel, Cherry ☛ Serving size= 1 piece, 64 g; GI= 59 (Medium); GL= 16.2 (Medium); Net carb= 27.5 g

Strudel, Peach ☛ Serving size= 1 piece, 64 g; GI= 59 (Medium); GL= 13.5 (Medium); Net carb= 22.9 g

Strudel, Pineapple ☛ Serving size= 1 piece, 64 g; GI= 59 (Medium); GL= 17.7 (Medium); Net carb= 30 g

# BEVERAGES

— **People with diabetes must avoid heavy drinking**

Cola From Fast-Food ☛ Serving size= 8 fl oz, 266 g; GI= 63 (Medium); GL= 16 (Medium); Net carb= 25.4 g

Cranberry Juice Cocktail, From Concentrate, Made With Water ☛ Serving size= 8 fl oz, 266 g; GI= 59 (Medium); GL= 18.5 (Medium); Net carb= 31.4 g

Energy Drink, Red Bull ☛ Serving size= 8 fl oz, 266 g; GI= 68 (Medium); GL= 18.5 (Medium); Net carb= 27.2 g

Fruit Flavored Smoothie (No Dairy) ☛ Serving size= 8 fl oz, 266 g; GI= 68 (Medium); GL= 13.7 (Medium); Net carb= 20.2 g

Fruit Juice Drink, Citrus Carbonated ☛ Serving size= 8 fl oz, 266 g; GI= 68 (Medium); GL= 12 (Medium); Net carb= 17.6 g

Fruit Smoothie, Light ☛ Serving size= 8 fl oz, 266 g; GI= 77 (High); GL= 17.7 (Medium); Net carb= 22.9 g

Fruit Smoothie, With Whole Fruit And Dairy ☛ Serving size= 8 fl oz, 266 g; GI= 77 (High); GL= 17.7 (Medium); Net carb= 22.9 g

Lemon-Lime Soda ☛ Serving size= 8 fl oz, 266 g; GI= 68 (Medium); GL= 18.8 (Medium); Net carb= 27.7 g

Lemonade-Flavor Drink Powder Made With Water ☛ Serving size= 8 fl oz, 266 g; GI= 68 (Medium); GL= 12.5 (Medium); Net carb= 18.4 g

Lemonade, Frozen, Concentrate, White Made With Water ☛ Serving size= 8 fl oz, 266 g; GI= 68 (Medium); GL= 18.8 (Medium); Net carb= 27.7 g

Lemonade, Fruit Flavored Drink ☛ Serving size= 8 fl oz, 266 g; GI= 68 (Medium); GL= 11.8 (Medium); Net carb= 17.4 g

Pepper Soda ☛ Serving size= 8 fl oz, 266 g; GI= 68 (Medium); GL= 18.8 (Medium); Net carb= 27.7 g

# DAIRY AND SOY ALTERNATIVES

Cream, heavy, whipped ☞ Serving size: 1 oz (28.35 g); GI= 55.4 (Low); GL= 4.7 (Medium); Net carb= 8.5 g

Cream, whipped, (pressurized container) ☞ Serving size: 1 oz (28.35 g); GI= 55.4 (Medium); GL= 4.7 (Medium); Net carb= 8.5 g

Milk dessert, chocolate ☞ Serving size: 1 cup (136 g); GI= 61 (Medium); GL= 13.3 (Medium); Net carb= 21.8 g

Milk dessert, flavors other than chocolate ☞ Serving size: 1 cup (136 g); GI= 61 (Medium); GL= 13.3 (Medium); Net carb= 21.8 g

Milk dessert, flavors other than chocolate, reduced calorie ☞ Serving size: 1 cup (136 g); GI= 50 (Low); GL= 11.6 (Medium); Net carb= 23.2 g

Milk dessert, flavors other than chocolate ☞ Serving size: 1 cup (136 g); GI= 50 (Low); GL= 11.6 (Medium); Net carb= 23.2 g

Milk shake (average value) ☞ Serving size: 1 cup (226g grams); GI= 44 (Low); GL= 17.9 (Medium); Net carb= 40.7 g

Milk-based fruit drink ☛ Serving size: 1 cup (226g grams); GI= 42.5 (Low); GL= 19.2 (Medium); Net carb= 45.2 g

Milk, oat ☛ Serving size: 1 cup (245 g); GI= 105 (High); GL= 16.8 (Medium); Net carb= 16 g

Milk, rice ☛ Serving size: 1 cup (245 g); GI= 86 (High); GL= 19 (Medium); Net carb= 22.1 g

Mousse chocolate ☛ Serving size: 1 cup (120 g); GI= 69 (Medium); GL= 19.3 (Medium); Net carb= 28 g

Pudding, canned, With chocolate and/or non-chocolate flavors ☛ Serving size: 4 oz (120 g); GI= 44 (Low); GL= 10.6 (Medium); Net carb= 24.1 g

Pudding, canned, tapioca ☛ Serving size: 4 oz (120 g); GI= 64 (Medium); GL= 16.3 (Medium); Net carb= 25.5 g

Pudding, coconut ☛ Serving size: 4 oz (120 g); GI= 44 (Low); GL= 12.7 (Medium); Net carb= 28.9 g

Pudding, rice ☛ Serving size: 4 oz (120 g); GI= 54 (Low); GL= 15.1 (Medium); Net carb= 28 g

Pudding, rice flour, with nuts ☛ Serving size: 4 oz (120 g); GI= 54 (Low); GL= 15.1 (Medium); Net carb= 28 g

Pudding, tapioca, made with milk, from dry mix ☛ Serving size: 4 oz (120 g); GI= 63 (Medium); GL= 16.3 (Medium); Net carb= 26.1 g

Pudding, tapioca, made with milk, from home recipe ☛ Serving size: 4 oz (120 g); GI= 62.5 (Medium); GL= 16.3 (Medium); Net carb= 26.1 g

Pudding, with fruit and vanilla wafers ☛ Serving size: 4 oz (120 g); GI= 86 (High); GL= 15.4 (Medium); Net carb= 26.1 g

# FRUITS AND FRUITS PRODUCTS

Apple Fried ☞ Serving size= 1 cup, 179 (g); GI= 38 (Low); GL= 14.9 (Medium); Net carbs= 39.1 g

Apple Juice ☞ Serving size= 1 cup, 248 (g); GI= 59 (Medium); GL= 16.2 (Medium); Net carbs= 27.5 g

Apricots, Canned, Drained, without added sugar ☞ Serving size= 1 cup, halves, 219 (g); GI= 31 (Low); GL= 12.6 (Medium); Net carbs= 40.8 g

Blackberries, Canned Heavy Syrup ☞ Serving size= 1 cup, 256 (g); GI= 25 (Low); GL= 12.6 (Medium); Net carbs= 50.4 g

Blackberry Juice, Canned ☞ Serving size= 1 cup, 250 (g); GI= 61 (Medium); GL= 11.7 (Medium); Net carbs= 19.3 g

Cherimoya ☞ Serving size= 1 cup, pieces, 160 (g); GI= 59 (Medium); GL= 13.9 (Medium); Net carbs= 23.5 g

Cranberry Juice, unsweetened ☞ Serving size= 1 cup, 253 (g); GI= 59 (Medium); GL= 18.1 (Medium); Net carbs= 30.6 g

Fruit Cocktail, Or Mix Frozen ☛ Serving size= 1 cup, 215 (g); GI= 79 (High); GL= 16.1 (Medium); Net carbs= 20.4 g

Fruit Salad, (Peach + Pear + Apricot + Pineapple + Cherry), Canned ☛ Serving size= 1 cup, 245 (g); GI= 68 (Medium); GL= 11.4 (Medium); Net carbs= 16.8 g

Fruit Salad, Fresh Or Raw Without Citrus Fruits ☛ Serving size= 1 cup, 175 (g); GI= 53 (Low); GL= 11 (Medium); Net carbs= 20.7 g

Fruit Salad, With Citrus Fruit and Whipped Cream ☛ Serving size= 1 cup, 182 (g); GI= 51 (Low); GL= 11.2 (Medium); Net carbs= 22 g

Persimmon ☛ Serving size= 1 fruit, 168 (g); GI= 61 (Medium); GL= 15.4 (Medium); Net carbs= 25.2 g

Goji Berries Dried ☛ Serving size= 5 tbsp, 28 (g); GI= 63 (Medium); GL= 11.3 (Medium); Net carbs= 17.9 g

Grapefruit Juice ☛ Serving size= 8 fl oz, 240 (g); GI= 59 (Medium); GL= 10.5 (Medium); Net carbs= 17.9 g

Grapefruit Sections, Canned Juice ☛ Serving size= 1 cup, 249 (g); GI= 77 (High); GL= 16.9 (Medium); Net carbs= 21.9 g

Jackfruit ☛ Serving size= 1 cup, sliced, 165 (g); GI= 51 (Low); GL= 18.3 (Medium); Net carbs= 35.9 g

Kiwifruit ☛ Serving size= 1 cup, sliced, 180 (g); GI= 50 (Low); GL= 10.5 (Medium); Net carbs= 21 g

Litchis ☛ Serving size= 1 cup, 190 (g); GI= 50 (Low); GL= 14.5 (Medium); Net carbs= 28.9 g

Mangos ☛ Serving size= 1 cup pieces, 165 (g); GI= 51 (Low); GL= 11.3 (Medium); Net carbs= 22.1 g

Nectarine Cooked without added sugar ☛ Serving size= 1 cup, 262 (g); GI= 35 (Low); GL= 18 (Medium); Net carbs= 51.3 g

Orange Juice ☛ Serving size= 1 cup, 248 (g); GI= 69 (Medium); GL= 17.5 (Medium); Net carbs= 25.3 g

Orange Juice, From Concentrate ☛ Serving size= 1 cup, 249 (g); GI= 59 (Medium); GL= 16.5 (Medium); Net carbs= 28 g

Orange Sections, Canned In Juice ☛ Serving size= 1 cup, 204 (g); GI= 71 (High); GL= 14.2 (Medium); Net carbs= 20 g

Orange-Grapefruit Juice, Canned, unsweetened ☛ Serving size= 1 cup, 247 (g); GI= 69 (Medium); GL= 17.3 (Medium); Net carbs= 25.1 g

Papaya, Canned, Drained ☛ Serving size= 1 piece, 39 (g); GI= 72 (High); GL= 15.3 (Medium); Net carbs= 21.2 g

Papaya Dried ☛ Serving size= 1 strip, 23 (g); GI= 69 (Medium); GL= 11.1 (Medium); Net carbs= 16.1 g

Papaya Green Cooked ☛ Serving size= 1 cup, 244 (g); GI= 60 (Medium); GL= 13.4 (Medium); Net carbs= 22.3 g

Persimmons Japanese Dried ☛ Serving size= 1 fruit without refuse, 34 (g); GI= 71 (High); GL= 14.2 (Medium); Net carbs= 20 g

Pineapple ☛ Serving size= 1 cup, chunks, 165 (g); GI= 59 (Medium); GL= 11.4 (Medium); Net carbs= 19.3 g

Pineapple, Canned, Solids And Liquids, Water Pack ☛ Serving size= 1 cup, crushed, sliced, or chunks, 246 (g); GI= 79 (High); GL= 14.6 (Medium); Net carbs= 18.5 g

Pineapple Dried ☛ Serving size= 1 piece, 28 (g); GI= 69 (Medium); GL= 12.8 (Medium); Net carbs= 18.5 g

Pineapple Raw Extra Sweet Variety ☛ Serving size= 1 cup, chunks, 165 (g); GI= 59 (Medium); GL= 11.8 (Medium); Net carbs= 20 g

Plantains ☛ Serving size= 1 cup, sliced, 148 (g); GI= 40 (Low); GL= 17.9 (Medium); Net carbs= 44.7 g

Red Or Green Grapes ☛ Serving size= 1 cup, 151 (g); GI= 53 (Low); GL= 13.8 (Medium); Net carbs= 26 g

Tamarinds ☛ Serving size= 1 cup, pulp, 120 (g); GI= 23 (Low); GL= 15.8 (Medium); Net carbs= 68.9 g

Tangerine Juice ☛ Serving size= 1 cup, 247 (g); GI= 59 (Medium); GL= 14.4 (Medium); Net carbs= 24.5 g

Tangerines ☛ Serving size= 1 cup, sections, 195 (g); GI= 45 (Low); GL= 10.1 (Medium); Net carbs= 22.5 g

# GRAINS AND PASTA

Buckwheat Groats, Cooked ☛ Serving size= 1 cup (170 g); GI= 55 (Medium); GL= 15.3 (Medium); Net carb= 27.9 g

Congee ☛ Serving size= 1 cup (249 g); GI= 73 (High); GL= 12.8 (Medium); Net carb= 17.6 g

Fusili Cooked, made with durum wheat flour ☛ Serving size= 2 oz (57 g); GI= 61 (Medium); GL= 11.8 (Medium); Net carb= 19.4 g

Japanese Soba Noodles, Dry ☛ Serving size= 2 oz (57 g); GI= 41 (Low); GL= 17.4 (Medium); Net carb= 42.5 g

Kamut Cooked ☛ Serving size= 1 cup (172 g); GI= 40 (Low); GL= 16 (Medium); Net carb= 40.1 g

Macaroni cooked, made with wheat ☛ Serving size= 2 oz (57 g); GI= 61 (Medium); GL= 11.8 (Medium); Net carb= 19.4 g

Noodles Cooked made with Corn, (Gluten Free) ☛ Serving size= 1 cup (140 g); GI= 55 (Medium); GL= 17.8 (Medium); Net carb= 32.4 g

Noodles Cooked, Vegetable ☛ Serving size= 1 cup (160 g); GI= 49 (Low); GL= 17.1 (Medium); Net carb= 34.9 g

Oatmeal Cooked ☛ Serving size= 1 cup (234 g); GI= 51 (Low); GL= 12.3 (Medium); Net carb= 24.1 g

Pasta Cooked, made with wheat flour ☛ Serving size= 2 oz (57 g); GI= 73 (High); GL= 14.1 (Medium); Net carb= 19.4 g

Pasta Cooked, Prepared with Vegetable ☛ Serving size= 1 cup (140 g); GI= 51 (Low); GL= 15.9 (Medium); Net carb= 31.2 g

Pasta Cooked, Made with Durum Wheat and Whole Wheat ☛ Serving size= 2 oz (57 g); GI= 53 (Low); GL= 10.3 (Medium); Net carb= 19.4 g

Penne Cooked, made with durum wheat ☛ Serving size= 2 oz (57 g); GI= 59 (Medium); GL= 11.4 (Medium); Net carb= 19.4 g

Quinoa Cooked ☛ Serving size= 1 cup (170 g); GI= 50 (Low); GL= 14.9 (Medium); Net carb= 29.8 g

Rice Bran Cooked ☛ Serving size= 1 cup (118 g); GI= 33 (Low); GL= 11.2 (Medium); Net carb= 33.9 g

Rice Brown, Parboiled Cooked ☛ Serving size= 1 cup (155 g); GI= 38 (Low); GL= 17.5 (Medium); Net carb= 45.9 g

Rice Wild 100% Cooked ☛ Serving size= 1 cup (164 g); GI= 45 (Low); GL= 14 (Medium); Net carb= 31.1 g

Spaghetti Cooked, made with 100% whole wheat ☛ Serving size= 2 oz (57 g); GI= 35 (Low); GL= 11.9 (Medium); Net carb= 34 g

Teff Cooked ☛ Serving size= 1 cup (252 g); GI= 36 (Low); GL= 15.5 (Medium); Net carb= 43 g

Wild Rice Cooked ☛ Serving size= 1 cup (164 g); GI= 57 (Medium); GL= 18.3 (Medium); Net carb= 32 g

# VEGETABLES

Corn Cooked ☛ GI= 48 (Low); Serving size= 1 cup (169 g); GL= 13.3 (Medium); Net carb= 27.6 g

Corn White, From Canned, Cooked ☛ GI= 55 (Medium); Serving size= 1 cup kernels (169 g); GL= 11.5 (Medium); Net carb= 21 g

Corn Yellow And White, Cooked From Canned ☛ GI= 59 (Medium); Serving size= 1 cup (169 g); GL= 12.1 (Medium); Net carb= 20.6 g

Corn Yellow, Cooked From Canned ☛ GI= 62 (Medium); Serving size= 1 cup (164 g); GL= 12.9 (Medium); Net carb= 20.8 g

Corn Yellow, Cooked From Fresh ☛ GI= 62 (Medium); Serving size= 1 cup (154 g); GL= 18.8 (Medium); Net carb= 30.4 g

Dasheen, boiled ☛ GI= 32 (Low); Serving size= 1 cup, pieces (142 g); GL= 13.3 (Medium); Net carb= 41.6 g

Lentil Sprouts ☛ GI= 32 (Low); Serving size= 1 cup (170 g); GL= 12 (Medium); Net carb= 37.6 g

Onion Rings, Fried or Batter-Dipped Baked, From Fresh ☛ GI= 95

(High); Serving size= 10 small rings (48 g); GL= 13.7 (Medium); Net carb= 14.4 g

Palm Hearts, Cooked ☛ GI= 38 (Low); Serving size= 1 cup (146 g); GL= 13.3 (Medium); Net carb= 35 g

Parsnips Creamed ☛ GI= 48 (Low); Serving size= 1 cup (228 g); GL= 12.5 (Medium); Net carb= 26 g

Rutabagas, Cooked ☛ GI= 72 (High); Serving size= 1 cup, mashed (240 g); GL= 19 (Medium); Net carb= 26.4 g

Sweet Pickled Cucumbers ☛ GI= 32 (Low); Serving size= 1 cup, chopped (160 g); GL= 10.3 (Medium); Net carb= 32.2 g

Sweet Potato Candied ☛ GI= 66 (Medium); Serving size= 1 piece (45 g); GL= 10.6 (Medium); Net carb= 16.1 g

Sweet Potato, Baked In Skin Flesh ☛ GI= 66 (Medium); Serving size= 1 medium (114 g); GL= 13.1 (Medium); Net carb= 19.8 g

Sweet Potatoes, Raw ☛ GI= 66 (Medium); Serving size= 1 cup, cubes (133 g); GL= 15 (Medium); Net carb= 22.8 g

Taro Baked ☛ GI= 32 (Low); Serving size= 1 cup (132 g); GL= 12.2 (Medium); Net carb= 38 g

Water Chestnut ☛ GI= 54 (Low); Serving size= 1 cup (158 g); GL= 13.1 (Medium); Net carb= 24.2 g

Yam ☛ GI= 51 (Low); Serving size= 1 cup, cubes (150 g); GL= 18.2 (Medium); Net carb= 35.7 g

# PART IX
# THE WORST FOODS TO EAT (HIGH GLYCEMIC LOAD FOOD)

# BAKED PRODUCTS

Basbousa ☛ Serving size= 1 piece, 82 g; GI= 63 (Medium); GL= 25.5 (High); Net carb= 40.5 g

Biscuit—Plain Or Buttermilk Dry Mix ☛ Serving size= 1 cup, purchased, 120 g; GI= 70 (High); GL= 51.5 (High); Net carb= 73.6 g

Bread—Chapati Or Roti Plain ☛ Serving size= 1 piece, 68 g; GI= 81 (High); GL= 22.8 (High); Net carb= 28.2 g

Bread—French Or Vienna Whole Wheat ☛ Serving size= 1 slice 1 serving, 48 g; GI= 95 (High); GL= 20.5 (High); Net carb= 21.6 g

Brioche ☛ Serving size= 1 piece, 77 g; GI= 91 (High); GL= 24.1 (High); Net carb= 26.5 g

Cake Or Cupcake—German Chocolate With Icing Or Filling ☛ Serving size= 1 regular cupcake, 75 g; GI= 55 (Medium); GL= 20.1 (High); Net carb= 36.6 g

Cake Or Cupcake—Fruit With Icing Or Filling ☛ Serving size= 1 regular cupcake, 75 g; GI= 55 (Medium); GL= 22.6 (High); Net carb= 41 g

Cake Or Cupcake—Nut With Icing Or Filling ☛ Serving size= 1 regular cupcake, 75 g; GI= 55 (Medium); GL= 21.8 (High); Net carb= 39.7 g

Cake—White Made From Recipe Without Frosting ☛ Serving size= 1 piece, 74 g; GI= 55 (Medium); GL= 22.9 (High); Net carb= 41.7 g

Cake—Yellow Enriched Dry Mix ☛ Serving size= 1 serving, 43 g; GI= 55 (Medium); GL= 19.1 (High); Net carb= 34.7 g

Cake—Yellow Made From Recipe Without Frosting ☛ Serving size= 1 piece, 68 g; GI= 55 (Medium); GL= 19.6 (High); Net carb= 35.6 g

Cobbler—Apple ☛ Serving size= 1 cup, 217 g; GI= 67 (Medium); GL= 51.7 (High); Net carb= 77.2 g

Cobbler—Apricot ☛ Serving size= 1 cup, 217 g; GI= 67 (Medium); GL= 49.4 (High); Net carb= 73.7 g

Cobbler—Berry ☛ Serving size= 1 cup, 217 g; GI= 67 (Medium); GL= 60 (High); Net carb= 89.5 g

Cobbler—Cherry ☛ Serving size= 1 cup, 217 g; GI= 67 (Medium); GL= 50.3 (High); Net carb= 75.1 g

Cobbler—Peach ☛ Serving size= 1 cup, 217 g; GI= 67 (Medium); GL= 53.4 (High); Net carb= 79.7 g

Cobbler—Pear ☛ Serving size= 1 cup, 217 g; GI= 67 (Medium); GL= 57.8 (High); Net carb= 86.2 g

Cobbler—Pineapple ☛ Serving size= 1 cup, 217 g; GI= 67 (Medium); GL= 52.3 (High); Net carb= 78 g

Cobbler—Plum ☛ Serving size= 1 cup, 217 g; GI= 67 (Medium); GL= 53.9 (High); Net carb= 80.4 g

Cobbler—Rhubarb ☛ Serving size= 1 cup, 217 g; GI= 67 (Medium); GL= 66.3 (High); Net carb= 98.9 g

CornBread—Muffin Stick Round Made From Home Recipe ☛

Serving size= 1 small, 66 g; GI= 73 (High); GL= 21.3 (High); Net carb= 29.2 g

Cornmeal—Dumpling ☛ Serving size= 1 cup, cooked, 240 g; GI= 75 (High); GL= 43.7 (High); Net carb= 58.3 g

Cream Puff Eclair Custard ☛ Serving size= 4 oz, 113 g; GI= 59 (Medium); GL= 24.4 (High); Net carb= 41.3 g

Crisp Apple Apple Dessert ☛ Serving size= 1 cup, 246 g; GI= 61 (Medium); GL= 43.8 (High); Net carb= 71.8 g

Crisp Blueberry ☛ Serving size= 1 cup, 246 g; GI= 59 (Medium); GL= 57 (High); Net carb= 96.6 g

Crisp Cherry ☛ Serving size= 1 cup, 246 g; GI= 60 (Medium); GL= 68.2 (High); Net carb= 113.6 g

Crisp Peach ☛ Serving size= 1 cup, 246 g; GI= 63 (Medium); GL= 56.6 (High); Net carb= 89.8 g

Crisp Rhubarb ☛ Serving size= 1 cup, 246 g; GI= 59 (Medium); GL= 59.9 (High); Net carb= 101.5 g

Doughnut—Chocolate Cream-Filled ☛ Serving size= 1 doughnut, 65 g; GI= 75 (High); GL= 19.4 (High); Net carb= 25.9 g

Doughnut—Chocolate Raised Or Yeast With Chocolate Icing ☛ Serving size= 1 doughnut ( 3 inch dia), 71 g; GI= 78 (High); GL= 27.9 (High); Net carb= 35.8 g

Doughnut—Custard-Filled With Icing ☛ Serving size= 1 doughnut, 70 g; GI= 79 (High); GL= 30 (High); Net carb= 38 g

Doughnut—Raised Or Yeast Chocolate Covered ☛ Serving size= 1 doughnut ( 3 inch dia), 71 g; GI= 77 (High); GL= 27.5 (High); Net carb= 35.7 g

Dutch Apple Pie ☛ Serving size= 1/8 pie 1 pie (1/8 of 9 inch pie), 131 g; GI= 55 (Medium); GL= 31 (High); Net carb= 56.3 g

English Muffins—Whole Grain White ☛ Serving size= 1 muffin 1 serving, 57 g; GI= 77 (High); GL= 20.5 (High); Net carb= 26.6 g

Muffin—Chocolate Chip ☛ Serving size= 1 muffin, 58 g; GI= 63 (Medium); GL= 19.5 (High); Net carb= 31 g

Muffin—English Oat Bran With Raisins ☛ Serving size= 1 muffin, 58 g; GI= 70 (High); GL= 19.3 (High); Net carb= 27.6 g

Pie Crust—Cookie-Type Chocolate Ready Crust ☛ Serving size= 1 crust, 182 g; GI= 59 (Medium); GL= 66.3 (High); Net carb= 112.4 g

Pie Crust—Cookie-Type Made From Recipe Vanilla Wafer Chilled ☛ Serving size= 1 cup, 129 g; GI= 59 (Medium); GL= 38.1 (High); Net carb= 64.6 g

Pie Crust—Refrigerated Regular Baked ☛ Serving size= 1 pie crust, 198 g; GI= 59 (Medium); GL= 66.7 (High); Net carb= 113.1 g

Pie—Apple Diet ☛ Serving size= 1 individual serving, 85 g; GI= 59 (Medium); GL= 21.4 (High); Net carb= 36.2 g

Pie—Banana Cream Individual Size Or Tart ☛ Serving size= 1 tart, 117 g; GI= 59 (Medium); GL= 20.7 (High); Net carb= 35 g

Pie—Berry, Individual Size Or Tart ☛ Serving size= 1 tart, 117 g; GI= 59 (Medium); GL= 26.6 (High); Net carb= 45.1 g

Pie—Blackberry Individual Size Or Tart ☛ Serving size= 1 tart, 117 g; GI= 59 (Medium); GL= 23.4 (High); Net carb= 39.7 g

Pie—Blueberry Individual Size Or Tart ☛ Serving size= 1 tart, 117 g; GI= 59 (Medium); GL= 25.5 (High); Net carb= 43.3 g

Pie—Chocolate Cream Individual Size Or Tart ☛ Serving size= 1 tart, 117 g; GI= 59 (Medium); GL= 24 (High); Net carb= 40.6 g

Pie—Chocolate Creme Commercially Made ☛ Serving size= 1 serving .167 pie, 120 g; GI= 59 (Medium); GL= 26.7 (High); Net carb= 45.2 g

Pie—Peach Individual Size Or Tart ☛ Serving size= 1 tart, 117 g; GI= 59 (Medium); GL= 26 (High); Net carb= 44.1 g

Pie—Pear Individual Size Or Tart ☛ Serving size= 1 tart, 117 g; GI= 59 (Medium); GL= 25.6 (High); Net carb= 43.4 g

Pie—Pudding Chocolate, Individual Size, With Chocolate Coating ☛ Serving size= 1 individual pie, 142 g; GI= 59 (Medium); GL= 34.3 (High); Net carb= 58.2 g

Pie—Pudding Flavors, Individual Size or Tart, Other Than Chocolate ☛ Serving size= 1 small tart, 117 g; GI= 59 (Medium); GL= 26.1 (High); Net carb= 44.3 g

Pie—Raisin Individual Size Or Tart ☛ Serving size= 1 tart, 117 g; GI= 59 (Medium); GL= 27 (High); Net carb= 45.8 g

Pie—Rhubarb Individual Size Or Tart ☛ Serving size= 1 tart, 117 g; GI= 59 (Medium); GL= 25.1 (High); Net carb= 42.5 g

Pie—Strawberry Cream Individual Size Or Tart ☛ Serving size= 1 tart, 117 g; GI= 59 (Medium); GL= 19.1 (High); Net carb= 32.3 g

Pie—Strawberry Individual Size Or Tart ☛ Serving size= 1 tart, 117 g; GI= 59 (Medium); GL= 23.9 (High); Net carb= 40.5 g

Pizza Cheese And Vegetables Gluten-Free—Thick Crust ☛ Serving size= 1 piece, nfs, 149 g; GI= 61 (Medium); GL= 21.4 (High); Net carb= 35.1 g

Pizza—Cheese And Vegetables Whole Wheat—Thick Crust ☛ Serving size= 1 piece, nfs, 149 g; GI= 62 (Medium); GL= 23.2 (High); Net carb= 37.4 g

Pizza—Cheese From School Lunch Medium Crust ☛ Serving size= 1 piece, nfs, 147 g; GI= 63 (Medium); GL= 24.4 (High); Net carb= 38.7 g

Pizza—Cheese Gluten-Free—Thick Crust ☛ Serving size= 1 piece, nfs, 132 g; GI= 63 (Medium); GL= 22.6 (High); Net carb= 35.8 g

Pizza—Cheese Whole Wheat—Thick Crust ☛ Serving size= 1 piece, nfs, 132 g; GI= 64 (Medium); GL= 24.5 (High); Net carb= 38.3 g

Pizza—Cheese With Fruit Medium Crust ☞ Serving size= 1 piece, nfs, 137 g; GI= 64 (Medium); GL= 25.3 (High); Net carb= 39.5 g

Pizza—Cheese With Fruit—Thick Crust ☞ Serving size= 1 piece, nfs, 150 g; GI= 64 (Medium); GL= 27.8 (High); Net carb= 43.4 g

Pizza—Cheese With Vegetables From Frozen—Thick Crust ☞ Serving size= 1 piece, nfs, 143 g; GI= 64 (Medium); GL= 26.4 (High); Net carb= 41.3 g

Pizza—Cheese With Vegetables From Restaurant Or Fast Food Medium Crust ☞ Serving size= 1 piece, nfs, 133 g; GI= 64 (Medium); GL= 24.3 (High); Net carb= 37.9 g

Pizza—Cheese With Vegetables From Restaurant Or Fast Food—Thick Crust ☞ Serving size= 1 piece, nfs, 149 g; GI= 64 (Medium); GL= 27 (High); Net carb= 42.2 g

Pizza—Extra Cheese—Thick Crust ☞ Serving size= 1 piece, nfs, 141 g; GI= 65 (Medium); GL= 27.3 (High); Net carb= 42 g

Pizza—No Cheese—Thick Crust ☞ Serving size= 1 piece, nfs, 124 g; GI= 73 (High); GL= 32.5 (High); Net carb= 44.5 g

Pizza—Rolls ☞ Serving size= 1 cup, 119 g; GI= 80 (High); GL= 49.6 (High); Net carb= 62 g

Roll—Sweet Frosted ☞ Serving size= 1 small, 54 g; GI= 77 (High); GL= 20.1 (High); Net carb= 26.1 g

Roll—Sweet With Fruit Frosted ☞ Serving size= 1 small, 54 g; GI= 77 (High); GL= 21.4 (High); Net carb= 27.8 g

Waffle—Chocolate Chip Frozen—Ready-To-Heat ☞ Serving size= 2 waffles, 70 g; GI= 76 (High); GL= 23.5 (High); Net carb= 30.9 g

Waffle—Whole Wheat Lowfat Frozen—Ready-To-Heat ☞ Serving size= 1 serving 2 waffles, 70 g; GI= 72 (High); GL= 22.6 (High); Net carb= 31.4 g

# BEEF, LAMP, VEAL, PORK & POULTRY

Beef-Offal—Heart: Breaded + fried 🖝 Serving size= 3 oz, 85 g; GI= 95 (High); GL= 20 (High); Net carb= 21 g

Beef—Bottom Round: Breaded + fried 🖝 Serving size= 3 oz, 85 g; GI= 95 (High); GL= 20 (High); Net carb= 21 g

Beef—Brain: Breaded + fried 🖝 Serving size= 3 oz, 85 g; GI= 95 (High); GL= 20 (High); Net carb= 21 g

Beef—Brisket: Breaded + fried 🖝 Serving size= 3 oz, 85 g; GI= 95 (High); GL= 20 (High); Net carb= 21 g

Beef—Chuck Roast: Breaded + fried 🖝 Serving size= 3 oz, 85 g; GI= 95 (High); GL= 20 (High); Net carb= 21 g

Beef—Chuck Steak Varieties Chart: Breaded + fried 🖝 Serving size= 3 oz, 85 g; GI= 95 (High); GL= 20 (High); Net carb= 21 g

Beef—Cuts of Steak: Breaded + fried 🖝 Serving size= 3 oz, 85 g; GI= 95 (High); GL= 20 (High); Net carb= 21 g

Beef—Delmonico Steak: Breaded + fried 🖝 Serving size= 3 oz, 85 g; GI= 95 (High); GL= 20 (High); Net carb= 21 g

Beef—Hanger Steak: Breaded + fried ☞ Serving size= 3 oz, 85 g; GI= 95 (High); GL= 20 (High); Net carb= 21 g

Beef—Kidney: Breaded + fried ☞ Serving size= 1 slice, 81 g; GI= 95 (High); GL= 20 (High); Net carb= 21 g

Beef—Liver: Battered + fried ☞ Serving size= 1 slice, 81 g; GI= 95 (High); GL= 20 (High); Net carb= 21.1 g

Beef—Liver: Breaded + fried ☞ Serving size= 1 slice, 81 g; GI= 95 (High); GL= 23.8 (High); Net carb= 25.1 g

Beef—Loin Steaks and/or Steak Types: Breaded + fried ☞ Serving size= 3 oz, 85 g; GI= 95 (High); GL= 20 (High); Net carb= 21 g

Beef—Mock Tender Petite Fillet: Breaded + fried ☞ Serving size= 3 oz, 85 g; GI= 95 (High); GL= 20 (High); Net carb= 21 g

Beef—Prime Rib: Breaded + fried ☞ Serving size= 3 oz, 85 g; GI= 95 (High); GL= 20 (High); Net carb= 21 g

Beef—Rib Steak Cuts: Breaded + fried ☞ Serving size= 3 oz, 85 g; GI= 95 (High); GL= 20 (High); Net carb= 21 g

Beef—Round Steak Varieties: Breaded + fried ☞ Serving size= 3 oz, 85 g; GI= 95 (High); GL= 20 (High); Net carb= 21 g

Beef—Short Loin: Breaded + fried ☞ Serving size= 3 oz, 85 g; GI= 95 (High); GL= 20 (High); Net carb= 21 g

Beef—Short Ribs: Breaded + fried ☞ Serving size= 3 oz, 85 g; GI= 95 (High); GL= 20 (High); Net carb= 21 g

Beef—T-Bone Steak: Breaded + fried ☞ Serving size= 3 oz, 85 g; GI= 95 (High); GL= 20 (High); Net carb= 21 g

Beef—Tenderloin: Breaded + fried ☞ Serving size= 3 oz, 85 g; GI= 95 (High); GL= 20 (High); Net carb= 21 g

Beef—Tongue: Breaded + fried ☞ Serving size= 1 slice, 81 g; GI= 95 (High); GL= 20 (High); Net carb= 21 g

Beef—Top Sirloin: Breaded + fried ☞ Serving size= 3 oz, 85 g; GI= 95 (High); GL= 20 (High); Net carb= 21 g

Beef—Tri-Tip: Breaded + fried ☞ Serving size= 3 oz, 85 g; GI= 95 (High); GL= 20 (High); Net carb= 21 g

Beef—Tripe: Breaded + fried ☞ Serving size= 1 slice, 81 g; GI= 95 (High); GL= 20 (High); Net carb= 21 g

Chicken—Backs and Necks: Breaded + fried ☞ Serving size= 3 oz, 85 g; GI= 95 (High); GL= 20 (High); Net carb= 21 g

Chicken—Breast Fillet Tenderloin: Breaded + fried ☞ Serving size= 3 oz, 85 g; GI= 95 (High); GL= 20 (High); Net carb= 21 g

Chicken—Drumstick: Breaded + fried ☞ Serving size= 3 oz, 85 g; GI= 95 (High); GL= 20 (High); Net carb= 21 g

Chicken—Leg: Breaded + fried ☞ Serving size= 3 oz, 85 g; GI= 95 (High); GL= 20 (High); Net carb= 21 g

Chicken—Tender: Breaded + fried ☞ Serving size= 3 oz, 85 g; GI= 95 (High); GL= 20 (High); Net carb= 21 g

Chicken—Thigh: Breaded + fried ☞ Serving size= 3 oz, 85 g; GI= 95 (High); GL= 20 (High); Net carb= 21 g

Chicken—Wing: Breaded + fried ☞ Serving size= 3 oz, 85 g; GI= 95 (High); GL= 20 (High); Net carb= 21 g

Lamb—Breast: Breaded + fried ☞ Serving size= 3 oz, 85 g; GI= 95 (High); GL= 20 (High); Net carb= 21 g

Lamb—Cutlets: Breaded + fried ☞ Serving size= 3 oz, 85 g; GI= 95 (High); GL= 20 (High); Net carb= 21 g

Lamb—Leg: Breaded + fried ☞ Serving size= 3 oz, 85 g; GI= 95 (High); GL= 20 (High); Net carb= 21 g

Lamb—Loin: Breaded + fried ☞ Serving size= 3 oz, 85 g; GI= 95 (High); GL= 20 (High); Net carb= 21 g

Lamb—Neck: Breaded + fried ☛ Serving size= 3 oz, 85 g; GI= 95 (High); GL= 20 (High); Net carb= 21 g

Lamb—Rack: Breaded + fried ☛ Serving size= 3 oz, 85 g; GI= 95 (High); GL= 20 (High); Net carb= 21 g

Lamb—Rump: Breaded + fried ☛ Serving size= 3 oz, 85 g; GI= 95 (High); GL= 20 (High); Net carb= 21 g

Lamb—Shank: Breaded + fried ☛ Serving size= 3 oz, 85 g; GI= 95 (High); GL= 20 (High); Net carb= 21 g

Lamb—Shoulder: Breaded + fried ☛ Serving size= 3 oz, 85 g; GI= 95 (High); GL= 20 (High); Net carb= 21 g

Pork—back ribs: Breaded + fried ☛ Serving size= 3 oz, 85 g; GI= 95 (High); GL= 20 (High); Net carb= 21 g

Pork—Belly: Breaded + fried ☛ Serving size= 3 oz, 85 g; GI= 95 (High); GL= 20 (High); Net carb= 21 g

Pork—Cutlets: Breaded + fried ☛ Serving size= 3 oz, 85 g; GI= 95 (High); GL= 20 (High); Net carb= 21 g

Pork—Garlic Sausages: Breaded + fried ☛ Serving size= 3 oz, 85 g; GI= 95 (High); GL= 20 (High); Net carb= 21 g

Pork—Ham: Breaded + fried ☛ Serving size= 3 oz, 85 g; GI= 95 (High); GL= 20 (High); Net carb= 21 g

Pork—Loin: Breaded + fried ☛ Serving size= 3 oz, 85 g; GI= 95 (High); GL= 20 (High); Net carb= 21 g

Pork—Rib chops: Breaded + fried ☛ Serving size= 3 oz, 85 g; GI= 95 (High); GL= 20 (High); Net carb= 21 g

Pork—Roasts: Breaded + fried ☛ Serving size= 3 oz, 85 g; GI= 95 (High); GL= 20 (High); Net carb= 21 g

Pork—Sausages: Breaded + fried ☛ Serving size= 3 oz, 85 g; GI= 95 (High); GL= 20 (High); Net carb= 21 g

Pork—Shoulder chops: Breaded + fried ☛ Serving size= 3 oz, 85 g; GI= 95 (High); GL= 20 (High); Net carb= 21 g

Pork—Sirloin chops: Breaded + fried ☛ Serving size= 3 oz, 85 g; GI= 95 (High); GL= 20 (High); Net carb= 21 g

Pork—spare ribs: Breaded + fried ☛ Serving size= 3 oz, 85 g; GI= 95 (High); GL= 20 (High); Net carb= 21 g

Turkey—Backs and Necks: Breaded + fried ☛ Serving size= 3 oz, 85 g; GI= 95 (High); GL= 20 (High); Net carb= 21 g

Turkey—Breast Fillet Tenderloin: Breaded + fried ☛ Serving size= 3 oz, 85 g; GI= 95 (High); GL= 20 (High); Net carb= 21 g

Turkey—Breast: Breaded + fried ☛ Serving size= 3 oz, 85 g; GI= 95 (High); GL= 20 (High); Net carb= 21 g

Turkey—Drumstick: Breaded + fried ☛ Serving size= 3 oz, 85 g; GI= 95 (High); GL= 20 (High); Net carb= 21 g

Turkey—Leg: Breaded + fried ☛ Serving size= 3 oz, 85 g; GI= 95 (High); GL= 20 (High); Net carb= 21 g

Turkey—Tender: Breaded + fried ☛ Serving size= 3 oz, 85 g; GI= 95 (High); GL= 20 (High); Net carb= 21 g

Turkey—Thigh: Breaded + fried ☛ Serving size= 3 oz, 85 g; GI= 95 (High); GL= 20 (High); Net carb= 21 g

Turkey—Wing: Breaded + fried ☛ Serving size= 3 oz, 85 g; GI= 95 (High); GL= 20 (High); Net carb= 21 g

Veal-Offal—Heart: Breaded + fried ☛ Serving size= 3 oz, 85 g; GI= 95 (High); GL= 20 (High); Net carb= 21 g

Veal—Bottom Round: Breaded + fried ☛ Serving size= 3 oz, 85 g; GI= 95 (High); GL= 20 (High); Net carb= 21 g

Veal—Brain: Breaded + fried ☛ Serving size= 3 oz, 85 g; GI= 95 (High); GL= 20 (High); Net carb= 21 g

Veal—Brisket: Breaded + fried ☞ Serving size= 3 oz, 85 g; GI= 95 (High); GL= 20 (High); Net carb= 21 g

Veal—Chuck Roast: Breaded + fried ☞ Serving size= 3 oz, 85 g; GI= 95 (High); GL= 20 (High); Net carb= 21 g

Veal—Chuck Steak Varieties Chart: Breaded + fried ☞ Serving size= 3 oz, 85 g; GI= 95 (High); GL= 20 (High); Net carb= 21 g

Veal—Cuts of Steak: Breaded + fried ☞ Serving size= 3 oz, 85 g; GI= 95 (High); GL= 20 (High); Net carb= 21 g

Veal—Delmonico Steak: Breaded + fried ☞ Serving size= 3 oz, 85 g; GI= 95 (High); GL= 20 (High); Net carb= 21 g

Veal—Hanger Steak: Breaded + fried ☞ Serving size= 3 oz, 85 g; GI= 95 (High); GL= 20 (High); Net carb= 21 g

Veal—Kidney: Breaded + fried ☞ Serving size= 2 slice, 81 g; GI= 95 (High); GL= 20 (High); Net carb= 21 g

Veal—Liver: Battered + fried ☞ Serving size= 1 slice, 81 g; GI= 95 (High); GL= 20 (High); Net carb= 21.1 g

Veal—Liver: Breaded + fried ☞ Serving size= 1 slice, 81 g; GI= 95 (High); GL= 23.8 (High); Net carb= 25.1 g

Veal—Loin Steaks and/or Steak Types: Breaded + fried ☞ Serving size= 3 oz, 85 g; GI= 95 (High); GL= 20 (High); Net carb= 21 g

Veal—Mock Tender Petite Fillet: Breaded + fried ☞ Serving size= 3 oz, 85 g; GI= 95 (High); GL= 20 (High); Net carb= 21 g

Veal—Prime Rib: Breaded + fried ☞ Serving size= 3 oz, 85 g; GI= 95 (High); GL= 20 (High); Net carb= 21 g

Veal—Rib Steak Cuts: Breaded + fried ☞ Serving size= 3 oz, 85 g; GI= 95 (High); GL= 20 (High); Net carb= 21 g

Veal—Round Steak Varieties: Breaded + fried ☞ Serving size= 3 oz, 85 g; GI= 95 (High); GL= 20 (High); Net carb= 21 g

Veal—Short Loin: Breaded + fried ☞ Serving size= 3 oz, 85 g; GI= 95 (High); GL= 20 (High); Net carb= 21 g

Veal—Short Ribs: Breaded + fried ☞ Serving size= 3 oz, 85 g; GI= 95 (High); GL= 20 (High); Net carb= 21 g

Veal—T-Bone Steak: Breaded + fried ☞ Serving size= 3 oz, 85 g; GI= 95 (High); GL= 20 (High); Net carb= 21 g

Veal—Tenderloin: Breaded + fried ☞ Serving size= 3 oz, 85 g; GI= 95 (High); GL= 20 (High); Net carb= 21 g

Veal—Tongue: Breaded + fried ☞ Serving size= 1 slice, 81 g; GI= 95 (High); GL= 20 (High); Net carb= 21 g

Veal—Top Sirloin: Breaded + fried ☞ Serving size= 3 oz, 85 g; GI= 95 (High); GL= 20 (High); Net carb= 21 g

Veal—Tri-Tip: Breaded + fried ☞ Serving size= 3 oz, 85 g; GI= 95 (High); GL= 20 (High); Net carb= 21 g

Veal—Tripe: Breaded + fried ☞ Serving size= 3 oz, 85 g; GI= 95 (High); GL= 20 (High); Net carb= 21 g

# BEVERAGES

**— People with diabetes must avoid heavy drinking**

Malt Beer Hard Lemonade ☞ Serving size= fl oz, 335 g; GI= 100 (High); GL= 33.7 (High); Net carb= 33.7 g

Pina Colada Canned ☞ Serving size= 8 fl oz, 266 g; GI= 35 (Low); GL= 25.6 (High); Net carb= 73.2 g

Chocolate-Flavored Soda ☞ Serving size= 8 fl oz, 266 g; GI= 68 (Medium); GL= 19.4 (High); Net carb= 28.5 g

Chocolate Syrup Made With Whole Milk ☞ Serving size= 1 cup (8 fl oz), 282 g; GI= 57 (Medium); GL= 20.1 (High); Net carb= 35.2 g

Chocolate-Flavor Beverage—Mix For Milk Powder With Added Nutrients Made With Whole Milk ☞ Serving size= 1 serving, 266 g; GI= 77 (High); GL= 23.5 (High); Net carb= 30.5 g

Chocolate-Flavor Beverage—Mix Powder Made With Whole Milk ☞ Serving size= 1 cup (8 fl oz), 266 g; GI= 77 (High); GL= 23.7 (High); Net carb= 30.7 g

Citrus Fruit Juice Drink—Frozen Concentrate ☞ Serving size= 8 fl oz, 266 g; GI= 69 (Medium); GL= 73.4 (High); Net carb= 106.4 g

Cocktail Mix Non-Alcoholic Concentrated Frozen ☞ Serving size= 4 fl oz, 144 g; GI= 79 (High); GL= 81.5 (High); Net carb= 103.1 g

Cranberry Juice Cocktail ☞ Serving size= 1 cup, 271 g; GI= 59 (Medium); GL= 19.6 (High); Net carb= 33.2 g

Cranberry Juice Cocktail Bottled ☞ Serving size= 8 fl oz, 266 g; GI= 59 (Medium); GL= 21.2 (High); Net carb= 36 g

Energy Drink ☞ Serving size= 8 fl oz, 266 g; GI= 68 (Medium); GL= 27.1 (High); Net carb= 39.9 g

Energy Drink Full Throttle ☞ Serving size= 8 fl oz, 266 g; GI= 68 (Medium); GL= 21.9 (High); Net carb= 32.1 g

Energy Drink, Amp ☞ Serving size= 8 fl oz, 266 g; GI= 68 (Medium); GL= 21.9 (High); Net carb= 32.1 g

Energy Drink, Monster ☞ Serving size= 8 fl oz, 266 g; GI= 68 (Medium); GL= 20.4 (High); Net carb= 30 g

Energy Drink, Rockstar ☞ Serving size= 8 oz, 266 g; GI= 68 (Medium); GL= 23 (High); Net carb= 33.8 g

Energy Drink, Vault Citrus Flavor ☞ Serving size= 8 fl oz, 266 g; GI= 68 (Medium); GL= 23.5 (High); Net carb= 34.6 g

Fruit Flavored Drink Less Than 3% Juice ☞ Serving size= 1 cup (8 fl oz), 238 g; GI= 68 (Medium); GL= 25.9 (High); Net carb= 38.2 g

Fruit Juice Drink—Greater Than 3% Fruit Juice ☞ Serving size= 8 fl oz, 237 g; GI= 68 (Medium); GL= 21 (High); Net carb= 31 g

Fruit Smoothie (average value) ☞ Serving size= 8 fl oz, 266 g; GI= 77 (High); GL= 21.4 (High); Net carb= 27.8 g

Fruit Smoothie—With Whole Fruit And Dairy ☞ Serving size= 8 fl oz, 266 g; GI= 77 (High); GL= 21.4 (High); Net carb= 27.8 g

Fruit Smoothie—With Whole Fruit No Dairy ☛ Serving size= 8 fl oz, 266 g; GI= 77 (High); GL= 23.3 (High); Net carb= 30.3 g

Fruit Smoothie—With Whole Fruit No Dairy Added Protein ☛ Serving size= 8 fl oz, 266 g; GI= 77 (High); GL= 22.1 (High); Net carb= 28.8 g

Grape Soda ☛ Serving size= 8 fl oz, 266 g; GI= 68 (Medium); GL= 20.3 (High); Net carb= 29.8 g

Horchata Beverage—Made With Milk ☛ Serving size= 1 cup, 248 g; GI= 45 (Low); GL= 21.5 (High); Net carb= 47.9 g

Horchata Beverage—Made With Water ☛ Serving size= 1 cup, 248 g; GI= 45 (Low); GL= 22.3 (High); Net carb= 49.6 g

Kiwi Strawberry Juice Drink ☛ Serving size= 8 fl oz, 266 g; GI= 68 (Medium); GL= 22.2 (High); Net carb= 32.6 g

Lemonada Limeade (Minute Maid) ☛ Serving size= 8 fl oz, 266 g; GI= 68 (Medium); GL= 24.9 (High); Net carb= 36.6 g

Lemonade (Minute Maid) ☛ Serving size= 8 fl oz, 266 g; GI= 68 (Medium); GL= 21.9 (High); Net carb= 32.1 g

Lemonade—Frozen—Concentrate—Pink ☛ Serving size= 8 fl oz, 266 g; GI= 89 (High); GL= 115 (High); Net carb= 129.2 g

Lemonade—Frozen—Concentrate—Pink Made With Water ☛ Serving size= 8 fl oz, 266 g; GI= 68 (Medium); GL= 19.4 (High); Net carb= 28.5 g

Lemonade—Frozen—Concentrate—White ☛ Serving size= 8 fl oz, 266 g; GI= 89 (High); GL= 117.4 (High); Net carb= 131.9 g

Limeade Frozen—Concentrate—Made With Water ☛ Serving size= 8 fl oz, 266 g; GI= 68 (Medium); GL= 24.9 (High); Net carb= 36.7 g

Oatmeal Beverage ☛ Serving size= 1 cup, 248 g; GI= 59 (Medium); GL= 22.5 (High); Net carb= 38.2 g

Orange Breakfast Drink—Ready-To-Drink ☛ Serving size= 8 fl oz, 266 g; GI= 68 (Medium); GL= 23.7 (High); Net carb= 34.8 g

Orange Drink—Breakfast Type With Juice And Pulp Frozen Concentrate ☛ Serving size= 8 fl oz, 266 g; GI= 68 (Medium); GL= 70.4 (High); Net carb= 103.5 g

Orange Drink—Breakfast Type With Juice And Pulp Frozen—Concentrate—Made With Water ☛ Serving size= 8 fl oz, 266 g; GI= 68 (Medium); GL= 20.5 (High); Net carb= 30.1 g

Orange Drink—Canned With Added Vitamin C ☛ Serving size= 8 fl oz, 266 g; GI= 68 (Medium); GL= 22.3 (High); Net carb= 32.8 g

Orange Juice Drink ☛ Serving size= 8 fl oz, 266 g; GI= 68 (Medium); GL= 23.9 (High); Net carb= 35.1 g

Orange Soda ☛ Serving size= 8 fl oz, 266 g; GI= 68 (Medium); GL= 22.2 (High); Net carb= 32.7 g

Orange-Flavor Drink—Breakfast Type Powder Made With Water ☛ Serving size= 8 fl oz, 266 g; GI= 68 (Medium); GL= 22.7 (High); Net carb= 33.4 g

Orange-Flavor Drink—Breakfast Type With Pulp Frozen—Concentrate—Made With Water ☛ Serving size= 8 fl oz, 266 g; GI= 68 (Medium); GL= 22.1 (High); Net carb= 32.5 g

Strawberry-Flavor Beverage—Mix Powder Made With Whole Milk ☛ Serving size= 8 fl oz, 266 g; GI= 68 (Medium); GL= 22.2 (High); Net carb= 32.7 g

# DAIRY AND SOY ALTERNATIVES

Milk shake—with malt 🖙 Serving size: 1 cup (226g grams); GI= 53 (Low); GL= 21.6 (High); Net carb= 40.8 g

Milk shake—with malt 🖙 Serving size: 1 cup (226g grams); GI= 53 (Low); GL= 21.6 (High); Net carb= 40.8 g

Milk—condensed, sweetened, average value 🖙 Serving size: 1 oz; GI= 61 (Medium); GL= 11.2 (High); Net carb= 18.4 g

# LEGUMS AND BEANS

- **Eating raw or undercooked dried beans can lead to food poisoning**

Black Beans—Turtle Mature Seeds Raw ☛ Serving size= ½ cup, 150 g; GI= 41 (Low); GL= 29.4 (High); Net carb= 71.6 g

Broad beans (Fava)—Mature Seeds Raw ☛ Serving size= ½ cup, 150 g; GI= 40 (Low); GL= 20 (High); Net carb= 49.9 g

Chickpeas (Garbanzo)—Mature Seeds Raw ☛ Serving size= ½ cup, 150 g; GI= 36 (Low); GL= 27.4 (High); Net carb= 76.1 g

Cowpeas—Mature Seeds Raw ☛ Serving size= ½ cup, 150 g; GI= 50 (Low); GL= 37.1 (High); Net carb= 74.1 g

Green Peas—Split Mature Seeds Raw ☛ Serving size= ½ cup, 150 g; GI= 51 (Low); GL= 30.2 (High); Net carb= 59.1 g

Hyacinth Beans—Mature Seeds Raw ☛ Serving size= ½ cup, 150 g; GI= 49 (Low); GL= 25.8 (High); Net carb= 52.7 g

Kidney Beans—All Types Mature Seeds Raw ☛ Serving size= ½ cup, 150 g; GI= 37 (Low); GL= 19.5 (High); Net carb= 52.7 g

Kidney Beans—Red Mature Seeds Raw ☛ Serving size= ½ cup, 150 g; GI= 37 (Low); GL= 25.6 (High); Net carb= 69.1 g

Lima Beans—Large Mature Seeds Raw ☛ Serving size= ½ cup, 150 g; GI= 46 (Low); GL= 30.6 (High); Net carb= 66.6 g

Moth beans—Mature Seeds Raw ☛ Serving size= ½ cup, 150 g; GI= 51 (Low); GL= 47.1 (High); Net carb= 92.3 g

Mung Beans—Mature Seeds Raw ☛ Serving size= ½ cup, 150 g; GI= 42 (Low); GL= 29.2 (High); Net carb= 69.5 g

Navy Beans—Mature Seeds Raw ☛ Serving size= ½ cup, 150 g; GI= 39 (Low); GL= 26.6 (High); Net carb= 68.2 g

Pigeon Peas—Mature Seeds Raw ☛ Serving size= ½ cup, 150 g; GI= 31 (Low); GL= 22.2 (High); Net carb= 71.7 g

Pink Beans—Mature Seeds Raw ☛ Serving size= ½ cup, 150 g; GI= 37 (Low); GL= 28.6 (High); Net carb= 77.2 g

Pinto Beans—Mature Seeds Raw ☛ Serving size= ½ cup, 150 g; GI= 39 (Low); GL= 27.5 (High); Net carb= 70.6 g

Small White Beans—Mature Seeds Raw ☛ Serving size= ½ cup, 150 g; GI= 36 (Low); GL= 20.2 (High); Net carb= 56 g

Tofu Yogurt ☛ Serving size= 1 cup, 262 g; GI= 50 (Low); GL= 20.6 (High); Net carb= 41.3 g

White Beans—Mature Seeds Raw ☛ Serving size= ½ cup, 150 g; GI= 36 (Low); GL= 24.3 (High); Net carb= 67.6 g

Yardlong Beans—Mature Seeds Raw ☛ Serving size= 1 cup, 167 g; GI= 43 (Low); GL= 36.6 (High); Net carb= 85 g

Yellow Beans—Mature Seeds Raw ☛ Serving size= ½ cup, 150 g; GI= 36 (Low); GL= 19.2 (High); Net carb= 53.4 g

# FISH & FISH PRODUCTS

Clams—floured, breaded or battered AND baked or fried, baked ☞ Serving size= 3 0z (85 g); GI= 95 (High); GL= 11.9 (Medium)

Crab—soft shell, floured, fried ☞ Serving size= 3 0z (85 g); GI= 95 (High); GL= 11.2 (Medium)

Fish stick—patty, or fillet ☞ Serving size= 3 0z (85 g); GI= 95 (High); GL= 37 (High)

Fish stick—patty, or fillet, floured, breaded or battered AND baked or fried, baked ☞ Serving size= 3 0z (85 g); GI= 95 (High); GL= 37 (High)

Oysters—battered, fried ☞ Serving size= about 12 medium; GI= 95 (High); GL= 11 (Medium)

Oysters—floured or breaded, fried ☞ Serving size= about 12 medium; GI= 95 (High); GL= 11 (Medium)

Scallops—floured, breaded or battered AND baked or fried, baked ☞ Serving size= 3 0z (85 g); GI= 95 (High); GL= 13.7 (Medium)

# FRUITS AND FRUITS PRODUCTS

Apple Candied ☛ Serving size= 1 small apple, 198 (g); GI= 44 (Low); GL= 23.3 (High); Net carbs= 53 g

Apples, Canned in Syrup, Drained ☛ Serving size= 1 cup slices, 204 (g); GI= 89 (High); GL= 26.9 (High); Net carbs= 30.3 g

Applesauce, Canned in Syrup, Drained ☛ Serving size= 1 cup, 255 (g); GI= 89 (High); GL= 42.5 (High); Net carbs= 47.7 g

Apricot Dried Cooked Without Sugar ☛ Serving size= 1 cup, 270 (g); GI= 41 (Low); GL= 31.2 (High); Net carbs= 76.1 g

Banana, Baked ☛ Serving size= 1 banana (7-1/4 inch long), 128 (g); GI= 53 (Low); GL= 20.1 (High); Net carbs= 38 g

Banana, Batter-Dipped Fried ☛ Serving size= 1 small, 108 (g); GI= 53 (Low); GL= 21.3 (High); Net carbs= 40.1 g

Banana, unripe ☛ Serving size= 1 cup, mashed, 225 (g); GI= 45 (Low); GL= 20.5 (High); Net carbs= 45.5 g

Breadfruit ☛ Serving size= 1 cup, 220 (g); GI= 65 (Medium); GL= 31.8 (High); Net carbs= 48.9 g

Cherries Sour Red, Canned, Extra Heavy Syrup ☛ Serving size= 1 cup, 261 (g); GI= 73 (High); GL= 54.2 (High); Net carbs= 74.2 g

Cherries Sweet, Canned Extra Heavy Syrup Pack ☛ Serving size= 1 cup, pitted, 261 (g); GI= 73 (High); GL= 47.1 (High); Net carbs= 64.5 g

Cherries Sweet, Canned Juice ☛ Serving size= 1 cup, pitted, 250 (g); GI= 73 (High); GL= 22.5 (High); Net carbs= 30.8 g

Cranberry Sauce, Canned in Syrup, Drained ☛ Serving size= 1 cup, 277 (g); GI= 77 (High); GL= 83.8 (High); Net carbs= 108.9 g

Cranberry-Orange Relish, Canned in Syrup, Drained ☛ Serving size= 1 cup, 275 (g); GI= 77 (High); GL= 97.8 (High); Net carbs= 127.1 g

Dried Apples ☛ Serving size= 1 cup, 86 (g); GI= 45 (Low); GL= 22.1 (High); Net carbs= 49.2 g

Dried Apricots ☛ Serving size= 1 cup, halves, 130 (g); GI= 41 (Low); GL= 29.5 (High); Net carbs= 71.9 g

Dried Bananas ☛ Serving size= 1 cup, 100 (g); GI= 63 (Medium); GL= 49.4 (High); Net carbs= 78.4 g

Dried Blueberries (Sweetened) ☛ Serving size= 1/4 cup, 40 (g); GI= 73 (High); GL= 21.2 (High); Net carbs= 29 g

Dried Cranberries (Sweetened) ☛ Serving size= 1/4 cup, 40 (g); GI= 73 (High); GL= 22.6 (High); Net carbs= 31 g

Dried Figs ☛ Serving size= 1 cup, 149 (g); GI= 61 (Medium); GL= 49.1 (High); Net carbs= 80.6 g

Dried Peaches ☛ Serving size= 1 cup, halves, 160 (g); GI= 52 (Low); GL= 44.2 (High); Net carbs= 85 g

Dried Pears ☛ Serving size= 1 cup, halves, 180 (g); GI= 54 (Low); GL= 60.5 (High); Net carbs= 112 g

Durian ☛ Serving size= 1 cup, chopped or diced, 243 (g); GI= 49 (Low); GL= 27.7 (High); Net carbs= 56.6 g

Fig Dried Cooked With Sugar ☛ Serving size= 1 cup, 270 (g); GI= 83 (High); GL= 70.7 (High); Net carbs= 85.1 g

Figs, Canned in Syrup, Drained ☛ Serving size= 1 cup, 261 (g); GI= 82 (High); GL= 59.6 (High); Net carbs= 72.7 g

Figs Dried Stewed ☛ Serving size= 1 cup, 259 (g); GI= 61 (Medium); GL= 36.9 (High); Net carbs= 60.5 g

Fruit Cocktail (Grape + Cherry + Peach + Pineapple + Pear), Canned in Syrup ☛ Serving size= 1/2 cup, 130 (g); GI= 79 (High); GL= 22.4 (High); Net carbs= 28.3 g

Fruit Cocktai (Grape + Cherry + Peach + Pineapple + Pear), Canned in Syrup ☛ Serving size= 1 cup, 248 (g); GI= 79 (High); GL= 35.1 (High); Net carbs= 44.4 g

Fruit Cocktail (Grape + Cherry + Peach + Pineapple + Pear), Canned in Syrup ☛ Serving size= 1 cup, 237 (g); GI= 79 (High); GL= 20.3 (High); Net carbs= 25.7 g

Fruit Cocktail (Grape + Cherry + Peach + Pineapple + Pear), Canned in Syrup ☛ Serving size= 1 cup, 242 (g); GI= 79 (High); GL= 26.6 (High); Net carbs= 33.7 g

Fruit Cocktail, Canned Heavy Syrup ☛ Serving size= 1 cup, 214 (g); GI= 79 (High); GL= 28.9 (High); Net carbs= 36.6 g

Fruit Juice, Smoothie, Naked Juice, Mighty Mango ☛ Serving size= 8 fl oz, 240 (g); GI= 77 (High); GL= 27.7 (High); Net carbs= 36 g

Fruit Juice, Smoothie, Naked Juice, Strawberry Banana ☛ Serving size= 1 cup, 228 (g); GI= 76 (High); GL= 19.2 (High); Net carbs= 25.2 g

Fruit Salad (Apricot + Cherry + Peach + Pear + Pineapple), Canned in Syrup ☛ Serving size= 1 cup, 259 (g); GI= 68 (Medium); GL= 38.3 (High); Net carbs= 56.4 g

Fruit Salad (Banana + Guava + Pineapple + Papaya) Tropical, Canned in Syrup ☛ Serving size= 1 cup, 257 (g); GI= 68 (Medium); GL= 36.8 (High); Net carbs= 54.1 g

Golden Seedless Raisins ☛ Serving size= 1 cup, packed, 165 (g); GI= 53 (Low); GL= 67.1 (High); Net carbs= 126.6 g

Gooseberries, Canned in Syrup, Drained ☛ Serving size= 1 cup, 252 (g); GI= 78 (High); GL= 32.1 (High); Net carbs= 41.2 g

Grape Juice ☛ Serving size= 1 cup, 253 (g); GI= 66 (Medium); GL= 24.3 (High); Net carbs= 36.9 g

Grape Juice ☛ Serving size= 1 cup, 253 (g); GI= 66 (Medium); GL= 24.3 (High); Net carbs= 36.9 g

Grapefruit White Juice, White, Canned, sweetened ☛ Serving size= 1 cup, 250 (g); GI= 77 (High); GL= 21.2 (High); Net carbs= 27.6 g

Grapefruit Sections, Canned in Syrup, Drained ☛ Serving size= 1 cup, 254 (g); GI= 77 (High); GL= 29.4 (High); Net carbs= 38.2 g

Guanabana Nectar, Canned ☛ Serving size= 1 cup, 251 (g); GI= 63 (Medium); GL= 23.5 (High); Net carbs= 37.2 g

Guava Nectar, Canned ☛ Serving size= 1 cup, 251 (g); GI= 61 (Medium); GL= 23.3 (High); Net carbs= 38.3 g

Jackfruit, Canned Syrup Pack ☛ Serving size= 1 cup, drained, 178 (g); GI= 81 (High); GL= 33.2 (High); Net carbs= 41 g

Juice, Apple And Grape, Blend with added vitamin C ☛ Serving size= 8 fl oz, 250 (g); GI= 63 (Medium); GL= 19.3 (High); Net carbs= 30.7 g

Juice, Apple Grape And Pear, Blend with added vitamin C And Calcium ☛ Serving size= 8 fl oz, 250 (g); GI= 63 (Medium); GL= 20.1 (High); Net carbs= 31.9 g

Mango Nectar, Canned in Syrup, Drained ☛ Serving size= 1 cup, 251 (g); GI= 69 (Medium); GL= 22.2 (High); Net carbs= 32.2 g

Mangosteen, Canned In Syrup ☛ Serving size= 1 cup, drained, 196 (g); GI= 67 (Medium); GL= 21.2 (High); Net carbs= 31.6 g

Orange Pineapple Juice, Blend ☛ Serving size= 8 fl oz, 246 (g); GI= 66 (Medium); GL= 19.5 (High); Net carbs= 29.5 g

Papaya Cooked Or Canned In Sugar Or Syrup ☛ Serving size= 1 cup, 244 (g); GI= 72 (High); GL= 33.6 (High); Net carbs= 46.7 g

Papaya Nectar, Canned ☛ Serving size= 1 cup, 250 (g); GI= 72 (High); GL= 25 (High); Net carbs= 34.8 g

Peach Dried Cooked With Sugar ☛ Serving size= 1 cup, 270 (g); GI= 83 (High); GL= 58 (High); Net carbs= 69.9 g

Peach Nectar, Canned ☛ Serving size= 1 cup, 249 (g); GI= 81 (High); GL= 23.9 (High); Net carbs= 29.5 g

Peaches, Canned in Syrup, Drained ☛ Serving size= 1 cup, halves or slices, 262 (g); GI= 81 (High); GL= 53.2 (High); Net carbs= 65.7 g

Peaches Dried Sulfured Stewed With Added Sugar ☛ Serving size= 1 cup, 270 (g); GI= 83 (High); GL= 54.2 (High); Net carbs= 65.3 g

Peaches Dried Sulfured Stewed Without Added Sugar ☛ Serving size= 1 cup, 258 (g); GI= 52 (Low); GL= 22.8 (High); Net carbs= 43.8 g

Pear Dried Cooked Without Sugar ☛ Serving size= 1 cup, 280 (g); GI= 52 (Low); GL= 51.3 (High); Net carbs= 98.6 g

Pear Nectar, Canned ☛ Serving size= 1 cup, 250 (g); GI= 83 (High); GL= 31.5 (High); Net carbs= 37.9 g

Pears, Canned in Syrup, Drained ☛ Serving size= 1 cup, halves, 247 (g); GI= 83 (High); GL= 21.7 (High); Net carbs= 26.2 g

Pears Dried Sulfured Stewed Without Added Sugar ☛ Serving size= 1 cup, halves, 255 (g); GI= 52 (Low); GL= 36.3 (High); Net carbs= 69.9 g

Pineapple, Canned in Syrup, Drained ☛ Serving size= 1 cup, crushed, sliced, or chunks, 260 (g); GI= 79 (High); GL= 42.5 (High); Net carbs= 53.8 g

Pineapple Juice, Canned Or Bottled, unsweetened ☞ Serving size= 1 cup, 250 (g); GI= 79 (High); GL= 25 (High); Net carbs= 31.7 g

Pineapple Juice unsweetened ☞ Serving size= 1 cup, 250 (g); GI= 79 (High); GL= 24.6 (High); Net carbs= 31.2 g

Plantains Cooked ☞ Serving size= 1 cup, mashed, 200 (g); GI= 40 (Low); GL= 31.3 (High); Net carbs= 78.3 g

Plantains Green Fried ☞ Serving size= 1 cup, 118 (g); GI= 40 (Low); GL= 21.6 (High); Net carbs= 53.9 g

Plums, Canned in Syrup, Drained ☞ Serving size= 1 cup, with pits, yields, 183 (g); GI= 78 (High); GL= 30.9 (High); Net carbs= 39.6 g

Plums Dried (Prunes) Stewed With Added Sugar ☞ Serving size= 1 cup, pitted, 248 (g); GI= 79 (High); GL= 57 (High); Net carbs= 72.1 g

Plums Dried (Prunes) Stewed Without Added Sugar ☞ Serving size= 1 cup, pitted, 248 (g); GI= 50 (Low); GL= 31 (High); Net carbs= 62 g

Pomegranate Juice, Bottled ☞ Serving size= 1 cup, 249 (g); GI= 67 (Medium); GL= 21.7 (High); Net carbs= 32.4 g

Prunes ☞ Serving size= 1 cup, 132 (g); GI= 29 (Low); GL= 34.1 (High); Net carbs= 117.6 g

Prunes, Canned in Syrup, Drained ☞ Serving size= 1 cup, 234 (g); GI= 78 (High); GL= 43.8 (High); Net carbs= 56.2 g

Raisins ☞ Serving size= 1 cup, packed, 165 (g); GI= 59 (Medium); GL= 72.8 (High); Net carbs= 123.5 g

Raisins Cooked ☞ Serving size= 1 cup, 295 (g); GI= 61 (Medium); GL= 100.2 (High); Net carbs= 164.3 g

Rambutan, Canned in Syrup, Drained ☞ Serving size= 1 cup, drained, 150 (g); GI= 77 (High); GL= 23.1 (High); Net carbs= 30 g

Raspberries, Canned in Syrup, Drained ☛ Serving size= 1 cup, 256 (g); GI= 77 (High); GL= 39.5 (High); Net carbs= 51.4 g

Rhubarb, Canned in Syrup, Drained ☛ Serving size= 1 cup, 240 (g); GI= 77 (High); GL= 25.3 (High); Net carbs= 32.8 g

Shredded Coconut Meat (Sweetened) ☛ Serving size= 1 cup, 256 (g); GI= 77 (High); GL= 32.4 (High); Net carbs= 42.1 g

Starfruit Cooked With Sugar ☛ Serving size= 1 cup, 205 (g); GI= 77 (High); GL= 22.4 (High); Net carbs= 29.2 g

Strawberries, Canned in Syrup, Drained ☛ Serving size= 1 cup, 254 (g); GI= 75 (High); GL= 41.6 (High); Net carbs= 55.4 g

Tangerines, Canned in Syrup, Drained ☛ Serving size= 1 cup, 252 (g); GI= 59 (Medium); GL= 23 (High); Net carbs= 39 g

# GRAINS AND PASTA

Brown Rice ☛ Serving size= 1 cup (202 g); GI= 68 (Medium); GL= 32.9 (High); Net carb= 48.4 g

Buckwheat Groats Roasted Dry ☛ Serving size= 1 cup (164 g); GI= 55 (Medium); GL= 58.3 (High); Net carb= 106 g

Amaranth Cooked ☛ Serving size= 1 cup (246 g); GI= 95 (High); GL= 38.8 (High); Net carb= 40.8 g

Corn Grain White ☛ Serving size= 1 cup (166 g); GI= 55 (Medium); GL= 67.8 (High); Net carb= 123.3 g

Corn Grain Yellow ☛ Serving size= 1 cup (166 g); GI= 59 (Medium); GL= 65.6 (High); Net carb= 111.2 g

Cornmeal—Degermed Unenriched White or Yellow ☛ Serving size= 1 cup (157 g); GI= 68 (Medium); GL= 80.7 (High); Net carb= 118.6 g

Cornstarch ☛ Serving size= 1 cup (128 g); GI= 97 (High); GL= 112.2 (High); Net carb= 115.7 g

Couscous Cooked ☛ Serving size= 1 cup (157 g); GI= 65 (Medium); GL= 22.3 (High); Net carb= 34.3 g

Couscous Dry ☞ Serving size= 1 cup (173 g); GI= 65 (Medium); GL= 81.4 (High); Net carb= 125.3 g

Couscous Plain Cooked ☞ Serving size= 1 cup (160 g); GI= 65 (Medium); GL= 22.6 (High); Net carb= 34.7 g

Finger millet ☞ Serving size= 1 cup (174 g); GI= 104 (High); GL= 129.1 (High); Net carb= 124.1 g

Foxtail millet ☞ Serving size= 1 cup (174 g); GI= 59 (Medium); GL= 73.2 (High); Net carb= 124.1 g

Japanese Somen Noodles, Dry ☞ Serving size= 1 cup (176 g); GI= 41 (Low); GL= 50.4 (High); Net carb= 122.8 g

Kodo millet ☞ Serving size= 1 cup (174 g); GI= 65 (Medium); GL= 80.7 (High); Net carb= 124.1 g

Little millet ☞ Serving size= 1 cup (174 g); GI= 52 (Low); GL= 64.5 (High); Net carb= 124.1 g

Macaroni Vegetable, fortified Dry ☞ Serving size= 1 cup spiral shaped (84 g); GI= 50 (Low); GL= 29.6 (High); Net carb= 59.3 g

Millet Raw ☞ Serving size= 1 cup (200 g); GI= 53 (Low); GL= 68.2 (High); Net carb= 128.7 g

Noodles Cooked, made with Egg ☞ Serving size= 1 cup (160 g); GI= 55 (Medium); GL= 21.1 (High); Net carb= 38.3 g

Noodles Cooked, made with Rice, Dry ☞ Serving size= 2 oz (57 g); GI= 56 (Medium); GL= 25.1 (High); Net carb= 44.8 g

Noodles Cooked, Whole Grain ☞ Serving size= 1 cup (160 g); GI= 53 (Low); GL= 22.1 (High); Net carb= 41.6 g

Noodles, Cooked ☞ Serving size= 1 cup (160 g); GI= 55 (Medium); GL= 21 (High); Net carb= 38.1 g

Oat Bran ☞ Serving size= 1 cup (94 g); GI= 77 (High); GL= 36.8 (High); Net carb= 47.8 g

Pasta Cooked ☛ Serving size= 1 cup (140 g); GI= 63 (Medium); GL= 25.5 (High); Net carb= 40.4 g

Pasta Cooked, made with Brown Rice Flour, Gluten-Free ☛ Serving size= 1 cup spaghetti not packed (169 g); GI= 71 (High); GL= 36.6 (High); Net carb= 51.5 g

Pasta Cooked, made with Corn And Rice Flour, Gluten-Free ☛ Serving size= 1 cup spaghetti (141 g); GI= 71 (High); GL= 36.7 (High); Net carb= 51.7 g

Pasta Cooked, made with Corn Flour And Quinoa Flour, Gluten-Free ☛ Serving size= 1 cup spaghetti packed (166 g); GI= 70 (High); GL= 32.3 (High); Net carb= 46.2 g

Pasta Cooked, made with Corn, Gluten-Free, Dry ☛ Serving size= 1 cup (105 g); GI= 78 (High); GL= 55.9 (High); Net carb= 71.7 g

Pasta Cooked, Whole Grain ☛ Serving size= 1 cup (140 g); GI= 61 (Medium); GL= 22.2 (High); Net carb= 36.4 g

Pearl millet ☛ Serving size= 1 cup (174 g); GI= 54 (Low); GL= 50.7 (High); Net carb= 94 g

Rice Brown Cooked, Cooked Made With Oil ☛ Serving size= 1 cup (196 g); GI= 56 (Medium); GL= 25.5 (High); Net carb= 45.6 g

Rice Brown Cooked, Made With Butter ☛ Serving size= 1 cup (196 g); GI= 56 (Medium); GL= 25.5 (High); Net carb= 45.6 g

Rice Brown, Long-Grain Raw ☛ Serving size= 1 cup (185 g); GI= 51 (Low); GL= 68.5 (High); Net carb= 134.4 g

Rice Brown, Medium-Grain Raw ☛ Serving size= 1 cup (190 g); GI= 56 (Medium); GL= 77.4 (High); Net carb= 138.3 g

Rice White And Wild, Cooked ☛ Serving size= 1 cup (151 g); GI= 72 (High); GL= 21.9 (High); Net carb= 30.4 g

Rice White Glutinous Cooked ☛ Serving size= 1 cup (174 g); GI= 86 (High); GL= 29.9 (High); Net carb= 34.7 g

Rice White, Cooked Made With Butter ☛ Serving size= 1 cup (163 g); GI= 72 (High); GL= 31.4 (High); Net carb= 43.7 g

Rice White, Cooked Made With Oil ☛ Serving size= 1 cup (163 g); GI= 72 (High); GL= 31.5 (High); Net carb= 43.7 g

Rice White, Long-Grain Parboiled Cooked ☛ Serving size= 1 cup (158 g); GI= 67 (Medium); GL= 26.6 (High); Net carb= 39.7 g

Rice White, Long-Grain Precooked Or Instant, fortified Dry ☛ Serving size= 1 cup (95 g); GI= 56 (Medium); GL= 42.8 (High); Net carb= 76.4 g

Rice White, Long-Grain Regular Cooked ☛ Serving size= 1 cup (158 g); GI= 56 (Medium); GL= 24.6 (High); Net carb= 43.9 g

Rice White, Medium-Grain Cooked Unenriched ☛ Serving size= 1 cup (186 g); GI= 65 (Medium); GL= 34.6 (High); Net carb= 53.2 g

Rice White, Short-Grain Cooked ☛ Serving size= 1 cup (205 g); GI= 72 (High); GL= 42.4 (High); Net carb= 58.9 g

Rye Grain ☛ Serving size= 1 cup (169 g); GI= 59 (Medium); GL= 60.6 (High); Net carb= 102.7 g

Semolina Cooked ☛ Serving size= 1 cup (167 g); GI= 66 (Medium); GL= 76 (High); Net carb= 115.1 g

Sorghum Grain ☛ Serving size= 1 cup (192 g); GI= 66 (Medium); GL= 82.9 (High); Net carb= 125.5 g

Spaghetti Cooked, made with wheat flour ☛ Serving size= 2 oz (57 g); GI= 60 (Medium); GL= 20.4 (High); Net carb= 34 g

Spaghetti Cooked, made with white wheat ☛ Serving size= 2 oz (57 g); GI= 64 (Medium); GL= 21.8 (High); Net carb= 34 g

Spaghetti Cooked, made with whole wheat flour cooked ☛ Serving size= 2 oz (57 g); GI= 65 (Medium); GL= 22.1 (High); Net carb= 34 g

Spelt Cooked ☛ Serving size= 1 cup (194 g); GI= 55 (Medium); GL= 24.1 (High); Net carb= 43.7 g

Tapioca Pearl Dry ☛ Serving size= 1 cup (152 g); GI= 70 (High); GL= 93.4 (High); Net carb= 133.4 g

Triticale ☛ Serving size= 1 cup (192 g); GI= 79 (High); GL= 109.4 (High); Net carb= 138.5 g

Wheat Germ Crude ☛ Serving size= 1 cup (115 g); GI= 59 (Medium); GL= 26.2 (High); Net carb= 44.4 g

Wheat Hard Red Spring ☛ Serving size= 1 cup (192 g); GI= 93 (High); GL= 99.7 (High); Net carb= 107.2 g

Wheat Hard Red Winter ☛ Serving size= 1 cup (192 g); GI= 93 (High); GL= 105.3 (High); Net carb= 113.2 g

Wheat Hard White ☛ Serving size= 1 cup (192 g); GI= 93 (High); GL= 113.7 (High); Net carb= 122.3 g

# VEGETABLES

Cassava—cooked ☞ GI= 46 (Low); Serving size= 1 cup (206 g); GL= 34.1 (High); Net carb= 74.2 g

Corn Fritter ☞ GI= 65 (Medium); Serving size= 1 cup (107 g); GL= 26.9 (High); Net carb= 41.3 g

Corn, From Fresh, Canned or Frozen ☞ GI= 48 (Low); Serving size= 1 cup (256 g); GL= 20.7 (High); Net carb= 43.2 g

Corn Sweet White, Cream Style, From Canned ☞ GI= 52 (Low); Serving size= 1 cup (256 g); GL= 22.5 (High); Net carb= 43.3 g

Corn Sweet White, Canned or Boiled Whole Kernel ☞ GI= 52 (Low); Serving size= 1 cup (256 g); GL= 19.6 (High); Net carb= 37.7 g

Corn Sweet Yellow, Cream Style, From Canned or Boiled ☞ GI= 52 (Low); Serving size= 1 cup (256 g); GL= 22.5 (High); Net carb= 43.3 g

Corn White, Cream Style, From Canned or Boiled ☞ GI= 55 (Medium); Serving size= 1 cup (256 g); GL= 24.5 (High); Net carb= 44.5 g

Corn Yellow, Cream Style, From Canned or Boiled ☞ GI= 62 (Medium); Serving size= 1 cup (256 g); GL= 26.8 (High); Net carb= 43.3 g

Starchy Vegetables Including Tannier White Sweet Potato And Yam No Plantain ☛ GI= 84 (High); Serving size= 1 cup (190 g); GL= 48.8 (High); Net carb= 58.1 g

Starchy Vegetables Including Tannier White Sweet Potato And Yam With Green Or Ripe Plantains ☛ GI= 84 (High); Serving size= 1 cup (195 g); GL= 49.2 (High); Net carb= 58.6 g

Starchy Vegetables, Puerto Rican Style ☛ GI= 86 (High); Serving size= 1 cup (195 g); GL= 50.4 (High); Net carb= 58.6 g

Sweet Potato Canned ☛ GI= 66 (Medium); Serving size= 1 cup, pieces (250 g); GL= 30.3 (High); Net carb= 45.9 g

Sweet Potato Casserole Or Mashed ☛ GI= 66 (Medium); Serving size= 1 cup (250 g); GL= 25.7 (High); Net carb= 39 g

Sweet Potato Baked ☛ GI= 79 (Medium); Serving size= 1 cup, mashed (328 g); GL= 41.3 (High); Net carb= 52.2 g

White potato ☛ GI= 66 (Medium); Serving size= 1 medium (260 g); GL= 92.5 (High); Net carb= 15.8 g

White potato—baked, peel not eaten ☛ GI= 73 (High); Serving size= 1 medium (260 g); GL= 121.7 (High); Net carb= 19 g

White potato—french fries, breaded or battered ☛ GI= 75 (High); Serving size= 1 medium (260 g); GL= 117.1 (High); Net carb= 17.7 g

White potato—french fries, from fresh or frozen, deep fried ☛ GI= 75 (High); Serving size= 1 medium (260 g); GL= 111 (High); Net carb= 16.7 g

White potato, mashed, made with water, from dry mix ☛ GI= 85 (High); Serving size= 1 medium (260 g); GL= 135.3 (High); Net carb= 18 g

White potato mashed, from dry ☛ GI= 85 (High); Serving size= 1 medium (260 g); GL= 135 (High); Net carb= 18 g

White potato mashed, from fresh ☛ GI= 79 (High); Serving size= 1 medium (260 g); GL= 126 (High); Net carb= 18 g

White potato hash brown, from Fresh, Frozen or dry mix ☛ GI= 75 (High); Serving size= 1 medium (260 g); GL= 132.3 (High); Net carb= 20 g

White potato—home fries ☛ GI= 75 (High); Serving size= 1 medium (260 g); GL= 126.3 (High); Net carb= 19.1 g

# ABOUT THE AUTHOR

"Dr. H. Maher" is a joint pen name under which Dr. Y. Naitlho, PharmD, and H. Naitlho, MS/MBA, co-write books.

Dr. Y. Naitlho PharmD has over 25 years of pharmacy practice, applied nutrition research, and writing. He is currently a pharmacist and health and nutrition writer. He is the author of several books in the field of food science and human nutrition, and applied nutrition.

Dr. Y. Naitlho received his Doctor of Pharmacy from Perm State Pharmaceutical Academy. As a pharmacist and nutrition professional, He ensures that book design meets readers' dynamic learning needs and that content meets reliability and integrity standards.

H. Naitlho has over 30 years of engineering practice and science and engineering Research. He is the author of several books in the field of business management and coauthor of numerous books in food science and human nutrition, food engineering, and applied nutrition.

H. Naitlho holds an Engineering degree from the École Supérieure d'Aéronautique et de l'Espace (Sup'Aéro), an Engineering degree from the École de l'Air (Salon de Provence) and has an MBA from Laureate International Universities, a post-graduate degree in Automatics from Paul Sabatier University, and a further post-graduate degree in Mechanics from Aix Marseille University.

H. Naitlho brings the engineering mindset and scientific rigor. He consistently refines ideas, analyzes data, and carries consistency and a great sense of detail to their work.

Made in the USA
Las Vegas, NV
10 December 2023

82472652R00154